A Practical Guide on
Physiotherapy Assessment
for Physiotherapy Students

A Practical Guide on
Physiotherapy Assessment
for Physiotherapy Students

Gopal Nambi S
MPT PhD MBA (USA)
Assistant Professor
Department of Physical Therapy and Health Rehabilitation
College of Applied Medical Sciences
Prince Sattam Bin Abdulaziz University
Al-Kharj, Kingdom of Saudi Arabia

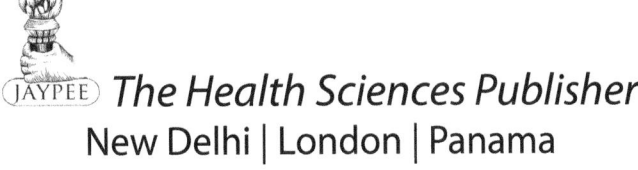

New Delhi | London | Panama

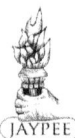
Jaypee Brothers Medical Publishers (P) Ltd

Headquarters
Jaypee Brothers Medical Publishers (P) Ltd
4838/24, Ansari Road, Daryaganj
New Delhi 110 002, India
Phone: +91-11-43574357
Fax: +91-11-43574314
Email: jaypee@jaypeebrothers.com

Overseas Offices

J.P. Medical Ltd
83 Victoria Street, London
SW1H 0HW (UK)
Phone: +44 20 3170 8910
Fax: +44 (0)20 3008 6180
Email: info@jpmedpub.com

Jaypee-Highlights Medical Publishers Inc.
City of Knowledge, Bld. 235, 2nd Floor, Clayton
Panama City, Panama
Phone: +1 507-301-0496
Fax: +1 507-301-0499
Email: cservice@jphmedical.com

Jaypee Brothers Medical Publishers (P) Ltd
17/1-B Babar Road, Block-B, Shaymali
Mohammadpur, Dhaka-1207
Bangladesh
Mobile: +08801912003485
Email: jaypeedhaka@gmail.com

Jaypee Brothers Medical Publishers (P) Ltd
Bhotahity, Kathmandu, Nepal
Phone: +977-9741283608
Email: kathmandu@jaypeebrothers.com

Website: www.jaypeebrothers.com
Website: www.jaypeedigital.com

© 2017, Jaypee Brothers Medical Publishers

The views and opinions expressed in this book are solely those of the original contributor(s)/author(s) and do not necessarily represent those of editor(s) of the book.

All rights reserved. No part of this publication may be reproduced, stored or transmitted in any form or by any means, electronic, mechanical, photocopying, recording or otherwise, without the prior permission in writing of the publishers.

All brand names and product names used in this book are trade names, service marks, trademarks or registered trademarks of their respective owners. The publisher is not associated with any product or vendor mentioned in this book.

Medical knowledge and practice change constantly. This book is designed to provide accurate, authoritative information about the subject matter in question. However, readers are advised to check the most current information available on procedures included and check information from the manufacturer of each product to be administered, to verify the recommended dose, formula, method and duration of administration, adverse effects and contraindications. It is the responsibility of the practitioner to take all appropriate safety precautions. Neither the publisher nor the author(s)/editor(s) assume any liability for any injury and/or damage to persons or property arising from or related to use of material in this book.

This book is sold on the understanding that the publisher is not engaged in providing professional medical services. If such advice or services are required, the services of a competent medical professional should be sought.

Every effort has been made where necessary to contact holders of copyright to obtain permission to reproduce copyright material. If any have been inadvertently overlooked, the publisher will be pleased to make the necessary arrangements at the first opportunity.

Inquiries for bulk sales may be solicited at: jaypee@jaypeebrothers.com

A Practical Guide on Physiotherapy Assessment for Physiotherapy Students

First Edition: **2017**

ISBN: 978-93-5270-064-6

Dedicated to
My loving Aunt
Late Pankajam K

Preface

As an academician, I noticed that there are many textbooks written on various treatment modalities in physiotherapy and the theories behind them, but the in-depth assessment of various specialities is still uncovered. Teachers and students had to refer to multiple books as no single book covered the practical assessment in detail. It led me to create a handbook *A Practical Guide on Physiotherapy Assessment for Physiotherapy Students* that did not fit into the mould offered by the existing textbooks. The book provides precise and concise explanation of all the content which is necessary for a strong foundation for practical and clinical assessments. At the same time, the contents of the book compiles and covers the practical curriculum of assessment in various universities. This book integrates different practical application procedures in physiotherapy which are often found split in many books. Hence, I hope to provide a better understanding in the field of practical physiotherapy.

This book was motivated by the desire to simplify the practical and clinical aspects of assessment in physiotherapy especially for the undergraduate and postgraduate physiotherapy students and clinical therapists working in the clinical set up. This book is referred from various national and international books to serve a number of objectives. One of the primary objectives is to define the different types of assessments commonly used in the field of health sector which provides the understanding of selection and application of different types of assessments in the field of physiotherapy.

With speciality assessment becoming increasingly important in a much wider ranges in the field of physiotherapy, therefore, the secondary objective is to discriminate the different speciality assessment (Orthopaedics, Sports, Neurology, Paediatrics, Cardio and Pulmonary, etc.) methods in the field of physiotherapy which provides the strong foundation in the speciality assessment.

Finally, a more pervasive objective is to expose all students and clinicians to not only use the assessment methods, but also to provide intellectual rich contents. I believe that, as times go on, all students and clinicians will take the benefit of this practical guide in a fruitful manner. As this book is still in its infancy stage, your feedback will be appreciated.

Gopal Nambi S

Acknowledgements

This work would not have been possible without the support of Dr Hamdan Ali Alshehri, Dean, College of Applied Medical Sciences, and Dr Fathy Elshazly, Head, Department of Physical Therapy, Prince Sattam Bin Abdulaziz University, Kingdom of Saudi Arabia. I am grateful to my friend Dr Walid Kamal and all the faculties and students those with whom I have had the pleasure to work with at CU Shah Physiotherapy College, Surendranagar, Gujarat, India.

I would like to express my special gratitude to my mentor and guide Dr MM Prabhakar, Medical Superintendent, Civil Hospital, Ahmedabad, Gujarat, whose stimulating suggestions and encouragement had always pushed me to do my best.

I would like to thank my mother Sujatha and brothers, whose love and blessings are with me in whatever I pursue. I also wish to thank my supportive wife Dr Dipika and my son Shaan, who provide me with unending inspiration.

Contents

1. Introduction to Assessment	1
2. Musculoskeletal Assessment	6
3. Orthosis Prescription Assessment	15
4. Prosthesis Prescription Assessment	23
5. Sports Injury Assessment	29
6. Sports Fitness Assessment	37
7. Neurological Assessment	43
8. Paediatric Assessment	52
9. Cardiac Assessment	59
10. Peripheral Vascular Disease Assessment	66
11. Respiratory Assessment	73
12. Intensive Care Unit Assessment	84
13. Geriatric Assessment	96

Annexures 105–136

1. General Medical History—Questionnaire	105
2. Type of Pain History—Questionnaire	106
3. Assessment of Range of Motion	107
4. Assessment of End Feel	110
5. Assessment of Capsular Pattern of Restriction	113
6. Assessment of Muscle Strength	114
7. Assessment of Muscle Length	116
8. Assessment of Sensation	117
9. Assessment of Reflex	118
10. Assessment of Non-equilibrium	119
11. Assessment of Equilibrium	120

12. Assessment of Dermatome	121
13. Assessment of Myotome	122
14. Assessment of Posture	124
15. Assessment of Gait	125
16. Assessment of Functional Activity	127
17. Assessment of Environment	129
18. Assessment of Cranial Nerves	130
19. Assessment of Disease Specific Scale	131
20. Assessment of Primitive Reflex	132
21. Assessment of Birth History	133
22. Assessment of Milestone	134
23. Assessment of Paediatric Muscle Strength	135
24. Assessment of Nutritional Status	136

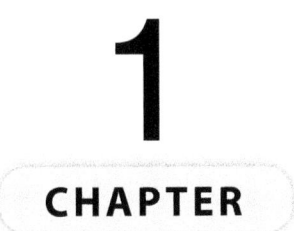

Introduction to Assessment
There is No Short Road to Knowledge

"Diagnosis arises from the examination and evaluation and represents the outcome of a process of clinical reasoning. This may be expressed in term of movement dysfunction or may encompass categories of impairments, functional limitations, abilities/disabilities or syndromes."

WCPT (1999, P.7)

CLINICAL DECISION MAKING

A thorough understanding of the patient and his/her disorder is a complex process which involves a series of interrelated steps which help the physical therapist to plan an effective treatment compatible with the needs of the patient and the goals of the health care team. These steps include:

1. Assessment of the patient.
2. Identifying the problem.
3. Determining the diagnosis.
4. Determining the prognosis and plan of care.
5. Implementing the plan of care.
6. Reassessment of the patient and evaluating the treatment outcome.

Adequate knowledge and experience, cognition process strategies, communication and teaching skills are important components of skilled decision making. Also a good communication amongst the rehabilitation team members and effective documentation is a must for timely reimbursement of the services.

PROBLEM-ORIENTED MEDICAL RECORD (POMR)

Originally developed by Weed, which is used by many therapists and institutions. Divides the treatment process in four phases.

Phase-1: Includes a detailed physical examination, laboratory and other tests and their results.

Phase-2: Interpreting the database to identify the specific problem.

Phase-3: Choosing a treatment plan for each of the problem also includes making of an evaluative progress note for each problem.

Phase-4: Assessment of the effectiveness of each of the plan and making necessary changes as the treatment progress.

SOAP Format

- **S**ubjective finding
- **O**bjective finding
- **A**ssessment
- **P**lanning of treatment.

Progress report is written in the subjective, objective, assessment and plan (SOAP) format. Subjective findings are what the patient or his/ her family report. Objective findings are what the therapist observes measures or tests. Assessment is correlating the subjective and objective findings to formulate long and short-term goals and plan is fixing the interventions.

The POMR highlights the relationship of the database to the treatment plan thus makes the specific problem of the patient to become the central focus of planning. To store the large amount of data computerized POMR is available.

ASSESSMENT AND EVALUATION

Assessment is the means of evaluating everything done during clinical decision making process (clinical reasoning). The effectiveness of a treatment is assessed by comparing the effects of the selected and processed techniques on the patient's signs and symptoms.

To complete proper assessment a thorough systemic examination is required. A correct diagnosis depends on knowledge of functional anatomy, accurate patient history, diligent observation and thorough examination.

ASSESSMENT OF THE PATIENT

It is believed that 80% of the information needed to identify the cause of the symptoms is given by the patient himself during history taking, thus making interviewing a very important skill for every physiotherapist to learn.

INTERVIEWING TECHNIQUES

1. Open-ended questions: Answers to these are in more than one word.
2. Closed-ended questions: Answer is either 'yes' or 'No'
3. Funnel technique or Funnel sequence: Starts with open-ended question and ends with close-ended questions.
4. Paraphrasing technique: Synthesizing and integrating the information obtained during questioning.

This helps in identifying the patient's problems. The resources available for proper intervention consist of three components:

1. Patient history
2. System review
3. Tests and measures.

   1. **Patient history:** History can be obtained from the patient, family or caregiver. Information obtained should contain the patient's primary complaint, history of present illness, significant medical condition that affected them in the past, lifestyle practices and habits.

      The therapist should listen carefully to the patient and observe for physical manifestations that reveal the emotional, state of the patient (e.g. Slumped body posture, poor eye contact, etc.).

      Interview is also an effective tool for establishing rapport for effective communication and mutual trust which in turn are vital for the success of the rehabilitation program.

   2. **System review:** It involves a brief examination of the entire body, followed by the detailed examination of the area of interest. This allows the therapist to decide if the patient's problems can be treated by him or if he should be referred to a specialist for significant medical condition.

3. **Tests and measures:** These are definitive assessment tools used to determine the degree of dysfunction (e.g. Range of motion, oxygen consumption, manual muscle test, etc.). Adequate training and skill are required to perform these tests to ensure the validity and reliability or it could result in inaccurate data leading to an inappropriate treatment plan. The therapist should review the patient's problem and choose for the appropriate test, also he/she should resist the tendency to gather extraneous data which might not only confuse the diagnosis but also increase the cost of care. Only in case where the initial data obtained are inconsistent should addition or specialized test be indicated.

PURPOSE OF ASSESSMENT

The purpose of assessment is to clearly understand the patient's problem. It serves several purposes.
1. Physiotherapy diagnosis.
2. Definition of physiotherapy objectives.
3. Determining treatment intervention.
4. Defining the parameters to monitor the effects of therapy.
5. Better recognize common disorder.
6. Impose overall health and functional outcomes.
7. Reduce vulnerability to subsequent illness.
8. Provide better quality of life.

FORMS OF ASSESSMENT

Different forms of assessment have described (**Maitland et al 2001**) and summarized as follows:
1. Assessment during initial consultation includes the welcoming and information phase.
2. Reassessment in various phases of each treatment session.
3. Assessment during the application of treatment intervention.
4. Retrospective assessment and prospective assessments to monitor the overall process.
5. Final analytical assessment including the parting phases in which measures are undertaken to enhance long tem.

Assessment at Initial Examination

At the first session the therapist has to gather information about the patient and accordingly draft a treatment plan. This information includes the following data.
- Biomedical
- Psychological
- Social
- Cultural

The key is to develop a clear, disciplined procedure of examination and planning. Improvisations are made to adapt the procedures for special needs of patients.

The following algorithm of information, procedures, reflections and planning are suggested for the first session - Algorithm of first session.

Within the first session the physiotherapist should collect information regarding:
- Causes and contributing factors for the condition.
- Treatment goals and suitable interventions.
- Activity involving the patient in the treatment process.
- Any precautions or contraindications in regards to examination or treatment procedure.

Reassessment

The term reassessment was first described in 1968 and now has become a part of the declarative knowledge of the profession (WCPT, 1999). The effect of any treatment needs to be continuously monitored and the treatment should be adapted as per the needs of the patient. Reassessment plays a key role in this process and it should be done during each treatment session.

- At the initial examination of the patient and after the examination of various active and passive movement tests.
- At the beginning of each subsequent sessions (pre-treatment assessment) to check for the effects of the last treatment session.
- Immediately after the application of treatment interventions. At the end of treatment session.

Purpose of reassessment: Allows the therapist to compare results proving the effectiveness of the treatment intervention selected.

Aids in differential diagnosis: Enables the physiotherapist to reflect on the decision made during diagnostic and therapeutic processes.

Reassessment helps the therapist to recognize patterns of clinical presentations with reactions to the interventions selected. Reassessment supports in the learning process of the patient.

Assessment during Treatment

The following factors are monitored during the treatment.

- Are the treatment objectives being achieved?
- Are there any undesirable side effects?

The physiotherapist needs to be alert for both the beneficial effects as well as side effects during intervention. As long as the changes are favorable, the technique may be continued. When changes cease to take place it is useful to perform a reassessment to evaluate the effect of the technique applied to the patient's condition.

Retrospective and Prospective Assessment

Retrospective Assessment

- This should include information from both the patient as well as the therapist.
- First information from the patient should be collected. Seek spontaneous information from the patient, as compared to 3 weeks ago how do you feel now?
- Effects of the treatment interventions: All the things done during therapy, do you think have been most helpful? Was any technique not helpful?
- What were the effects of the exercises recommendations and instructions given? Are there any difficulties in any of the self-management methods? Do they reach the expected goals?
- What have you learned from therapy so far?
- The symptoms and the level of activities have to be put in perspective to the period before the disorder had worsened.
- The therapist should check the treatment records for changes in the subjective and physical parameters after intervention.

Prospective Assessment

- After reviewing the therapeutic process, the treatment objectives for the next period of therapy should be decided.
- The following questions will help in planning.
    - On which aspects should we work together?

- Which activities need to get better? Are there any activities in your work or hobbies which you do not have the confidence to do or need to be very careful while performing? Which activities still need to get better you?
- If new treatment objectives have been defined (e.g. Pain during bending) then these activities are used as physical parameters during reassessment.

Final Analytical Assessment

- At the end of the therapeutic process a final assessment may be made. The process of this assessment is done over the last 2–3 sessions.
- The following information should be analyzed:
  - First examination.
  - Behavior of the disorder throughout treatment (Details derived from the retrospective assessment).
- State of affairs at the end of the treatment arises, taking into account the changes in subjective and physical parameters.

The patient and therapist together analyze:

- Overall therapeutic process: Which intervention brought which result?
- The learning process: What was especially important for the patient and has been learned?
- The effectiveness of any prophylactic measures and self-management interventions.
- Suggestions of any medical or other measures that can be carried out?

For the successful outcome the participation of the patient in planning is very essential. The timely reimbursement of the service can be provided. Patient participation in planning is essential in ensuring successful outcomes. Documentation is also an essential requirement for effective communication among the rehabilitation team members and for timely reimbursement of services.

CHAPTER 2

Musculoskeletal Assessment

SUBJECTIVE ASSESSMENT

Demographic Data

Name: _____ Date: _____

Age: _____ Sex: _____

Occupation: _____

Address:

Present: _____ Permanent: _____

Contact No.: Res _____ Off: _____

Referring Doctor: _____ Date of Next Visit: _____

Primary Diagnosis: _____

Case History

Chief Complaints: _____
_____
_____
_____

Past Medical History

Date of Onset: _____

Medical History: _____
_____
_____
_____

Medical History Questionnaire

1. What previous care has been sought for the problem?
2. Who else has treated the problem?
3. What tests and treatment did they perform?
4. What have you done to relieve the problem?
5. Has this problem occurred before? If yes, how was it treated or resolved?

    i. Previous Medications:

Medicine	Dosage	Frequency
(i) _____	_____	_____
(ii) _____	_____	_____
(iii) _____	_____	_____

    ii. Previous Surgeries:

Surgery Name	Date	Complication
(i) _____	_____	_____
(ii) _____	_____	_____
(iii) _____	_____	_____

    iii. Previous Diagnostic Test Reports:

    | X- Rays: _____ | C.T Scan: _____ | M.R.I: _____ |
    | Bone scan: _____ | EMG: _____ | Blood test: _____ |
    | Myelogram: _____ | Biochemical test: _____ | Others: _____ |

*General Medical History (Attached **Annexure-1**):*

Personal History

Do you use tobacco products? Alcohol? Recreational drugs? If yes,

Name and Frequency of cigarettes/day _____

Name and Frequency of Alcohol/day _____

Name and Frequency of Drugs/day _____

i. What percentage of your normal work activities are you able to perform?

   0%   10%   20%   30%   40%   50%   60%   70%   80%   90%   100%

ii. What percentage of your normal home activities are you able to perform?

   0%   10%   20%   30%   40%   50%   60%   70%   80%   90%   100%

iii. What percentage of your normal recreational activities are you able to perform?

0%   10%   20%   30%   40%   50%   60%   70%   80%   90%   100%

Family History
Family Background:
Hereditary complaint:

Occupational History
Related to present illness:
Occupational hazards for illness:

Social History
  i. Do you live alone and what type of work do you do in and outside of the home?
 ii. How has this problem affected your ability to perform your job?
iii. Do you have to climb stairs to get into your house? Reach the bedroom?

Economic History
1. Onset of Pain:
   a. Sudden: Yes/No, If yes, how? _____
   b. Gradual: Yes/No, If yes, how? _____
   c. Congenital onset: Yes/No, If yes, how? _____
2. Location of Pain (Through body chart)

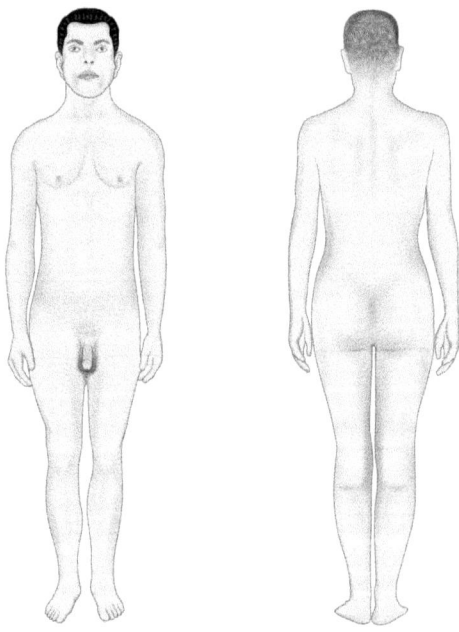

Has the pain change in location: Yes/No, if yes, where _____
Spread to other areas: Yes/No, if yes, where _____
Become more focused: Yes/No, if yes, where _____

3. Intensity of Pain (Ask the patient to rate his or her pain in this scale)
   Visual Analog Scale

No pain   Pain as bad as it could possibly be

4. Type of pain (Attached **Annexure-2**):
5. Behavior of symptoms:
   What makes your symptoms increase?
   i. Rest: yes/no, if yes which position _____
   ii. Activity: yes/no, if yes which position _____
   iii. Body position: yes/no, if yes which position _____
   What makes your symptoms decrease?
   i. Rest: yes/no, if yes which position _____
   ii. Activity: yes/no, if yes which position _____
   iii. Body position: yes/no, if yes which position _____
   Behavior of symptom during the last 48 hours:
   Better, worse, staying the same: _____

Recognizing Pain Patterns

Indicate a plus (+) for aggravating factors or a minus (-) for relieving factors

Liquor	Sleep/rest
Stimulants (e.g. caffeine)	Lying down
Eating	Distraction (e.g. television)
Heat	Urination/Defecation
Cold	Tension/Stress
Weather changes	Loud noise
Massage	Going to work
Pressure	Intercourse
No movement	Mild Exercise
Movement	Fatigue
Sitting	Standing

OBJECTIVE ASSESSMENT

Mental Status:

1. Level of Consciousness :
2. Orientation to
   i. Person :
   ii. Place :
   iii. Time :
3. General Arousal State :
4. Cognitive State :
5. Communication Ability :
6. Vital Signs:
   Blood pressure : 120/80 mmHg
   Respiratory rate : 16–20/min
   Pulse rate : 72–75
   Temperature : 98.6°F

Observation

General posture : _____
Ability to perform status: _____
Changing the position: _____
Transfer from sitting to standing: _____
Ambulate to the examining room: _____
Built of the patient: Ectomorphic/Mesomorphic/Endomorphic

Inspection

i. **Postural Alignment:**

   a. Anterior view:

Both eyes: _____	Acromion process: _____
Iliac crests: _____	ASIS: _____
Greater trochanter: _____	Patellae: _____
Ankle malleoli: _____	Waist angle: _____

   b. Posterior view:

Earlobes: _____	Spine of the scapula: _____
Shoulder: _____	Inferior angle of scapula: _____
Iliac crests: _____	PSIS: _____
Greater trochanter: _____	Buttocks: _____
Knee creases: _____	Ankle malleoli: _____
Spine: _____	

   c. Lateral view (see through the line of gravity – Impression) _____
   _____
   _____

ii. **Contour and Alignment of Bone and Joints:**

   Impression: _____
   _____

iii. **Size and Contour of Soft Tissue Structure:**

Soft tissue edema: _____	Joint effusion: _____
Muscle hypertrophy: _____	Muscle atrophy: _____
Muscle rupture: _____	Cysts, Rheumatoid nodules: _____
Ganglion: _____	Gouty tophi: _____

   Impression: _____
   _____

iv. **Size and Contour of Nails:**

   _____
   _____

   Clubbing (Grade): _____

v. **Colour and Texture of Skin and Tongue:**
   Cyanosis: _____ Pallor: _____
   Erythema (localized, generalized): _____ Yellow skin: _____
   Highly pigmented hairy areas: _____ Open wounds: _____
   Scars: New scar: _____ Old scar: _____
   Thickening, thinning, and hair loss: _____

Palpation

i. Bony Prominences (Pain, Abnormal Alignment):
   Antr surface: _____
   Postr surface: _____
   Lat surface: (Rt) _____ , (Lt) _____

ii. Soft tissue structures:
   Pain: _____ Tenderness (Grade): _____
   Swelling: _____ Spasm: _____
   Nodules: _____ Trigger points: _____
   Fascia tightness: _____ Mobility of soft tissue: _____
   Density and extensibility of soft tissues: _____
   Impression: _____

iii. Skin:
   Warmth: _____ Density: _____
   Extensibility of skin: _____ Peripheral pulses: _____
   Edema (pitting or non-pitting edema): _____ Grade: _____

Anthropometric Measurements

1. Limb length: (i) True length: (Rt) _____ (Lt) _____
              (ii) Apparent length: (Rt) _____ (Lt) _____
2. Circumference Measurement:
   Upper arm: Rt _____ Lt _____
   Forearm   : Rt _____ Lt _____
   Mid-thigh : Rt _____ Lt _____
   Calf   : Rt _____ Lt _____
   Chest   : _____

Examination

1. **Assessment of Range of Motion** (Attached **Annexure-3**):
   (Find the Amount, Quality, Pattern, Pain and Crepitus) AROM, PROM
   Impression: _____
   _____

2. **Assessment of End Feel** (Attached **Annexure-4**):
   (Feeling which is felt by the therapist as a resistance or a barrier to further motion)
   Impression: _____
   _____

3. **Assessment of Capsular Pattern of Restriction** (Attached **Annexure-5**):
   Impression: _____
   _____

4. **Assessment of Accessory Joint Motion:**
   (If passive ROM is limited or painful, assess the accessory joint motion in 1-6 grade)
   Impression: _____
   _____

5. **Assessment of Resisted Isometric Muscle Testing:**
   (Identify the problem in contractile or non-contractile structure – mention the muscle group)
   Impression: _____

6. **Assessment of Muscle Strength** (Attached **Annexure-6**):
   Impression: _____
   _____

7. **Assessment of Muscle Length** (Attached **Annexure-7**):
   Impression: _____
   _____

8. **Assessment of Hand-held/Isokinetic Dynamometry:**
   Impression: _____
   _____

9. **Assessment of Sensation** (Attached **Annexure-8**):
   Superficial: _____
   _____
   Deep: _____
   _____

10. **Assessment of Reflex** (Attached **Annexure-9**):
    Superficial: _____
    _____
    Deep: _____
    _____

11. **Assessment of Dermatome/Myotome** (Attached **Annexures-12 and 13**):
    Dermatome: _____
    _____
    Myotome: _____
    _____

12. **Assessment of Posture** (Attached **Annexure-14**):
    Impression: _____
    _____

13. Assessment of Gait (Attached **Annexure-15**):

Distance walked	Step length difference
Elapsed time	Cadence
Walking velocity	Width of walking base
Left stride length	Left foot angle
Right stride length	Right foot angle
Left step length	Right stride length to Right L.L length
Right step length	Left stride length to Left L.L length

Impression: _____

14. Assessment of Functional Activity (Attached **Annexure-16**):
Impression: _____

15. Assessment of Environment: (Attached **Annexure-17**):
Impression: _____

16. Special Test:
Impression: _____

17. External Devices Used:
Impression: _____

18. Other Systems Examination:
Nervous system:
CVS: DVT/ Postural Dysfunction/Edema:
Respiratory system: Type/ Pattern of breathing/ Chest expansion/ Chest deformities:
Skin: Pressure sore:
Bladder/ Bowel: Retention/ Constipation/ Autonomous/ Automatic bladder:
Sexual Function :
Physical Diagnosis :
Functional Diagnosis :

Professional Diagnosis:

Problem list: _____

Management

Short-term Goals

Aims : 1.
2.
3.
4.
5.

Means : 1.
2.
3.
4.
5.

Long-term Goals

Aims : 1.
2.
3.
4.
5.

Means : 1.
2.
3.
4
5.

Orthosis Prescription Assessment

SUBJECTIVE ASSESSMENT

Demographic Data

Name: _____   Date: _____

Age: _____   Sex: _____

Occupation: _____

Address:

Present: _____   Permanent: _____

Contact No.: Res _____   Off: _____

Referring Doctor: _____   Date of Next Visit: _____

Primary Diagnosis: _____

Case History

Chief Complaints: _____

Past Medical History

Date of Onset: _____

Medical History: _____
_____
_____
_____

i. Previous Medications:

Medicine	Dosage	Frequency
(i) _____	_____	_____
(ii) _____	_____	_____
(iii) _____	_____	_____

ii. Previous Surgeries:

Surgery Name	Date	Complication
(i) _____	_____	_____
(ii) _____	_____	_____
(iii) _____	_____	_____

iii. Previous Diagnostic Test Reports:

*General Medical History (Attached **Annexure-1**):*

Personal History

Family history:
Family Background:
Hereditary complaint:

Occupational History
Related to present illness   :
Occupational hazards for illness :

Social History
 i. Do you live alone and what type of work do you do in and outside of the home?
 ii. How has this problem affected your ability to perform your job?
 iii. Do you have to climb stairs to get into your house? Reach the bedroom?

Economic History
1. Onset of Pain:
   a. Sudden: Yes/No, If yes, How? _____
   b. Gradual: Yes/No, If yes, how? _____
   c. Congenital onset: Yes/No, If yes, how? _____
2. Location of Pain: (Through body chart)
   Has the pain change in location: Yes/No, if yes, where _____
   Spread to other areas: Yes/No, if yes, where _____
   Become more focused: Yes/No, if yes, where _____

Orthosis Prescription Assessment

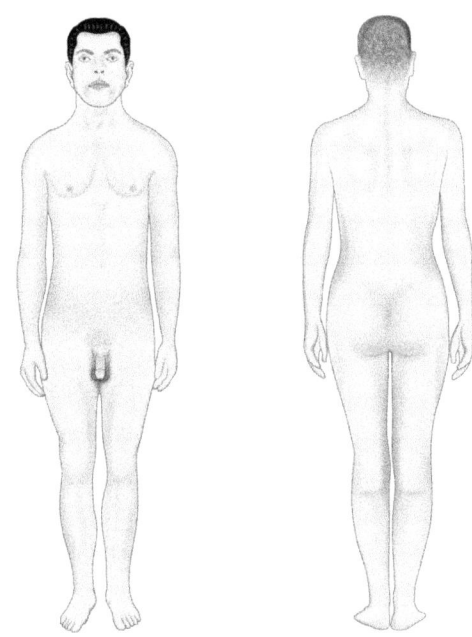

3. Intensity of Pain (Ask the patient to rate his or her pain in this scale):
   Visual Analog Scale:

   No pain   Pain as bad as it could possibly be

OBJECTIVE ASSESSMENT

Mental Status

1. Level of Consciousness :
2. Orientation to
   i. Person :
   ii. Place :
   iii. Time :
3. Vital Signs:

Blood pressure	:	120/80 mmHg
Respiratory rate	:	16–20 /min
Pulse rate	:	72–75
Temperature	:	98.6°F

Observation

General posture: _____
Ability to perform status: _____
Changing the position: _____
Transfer from sitting to standing: _____
Ambulate to the examining room: _____
Built of the Patient: Ectomorphic/Mesomorphic/Endomorphic

Inspection

i. **Postural Alignment:**
   a. Anterior view:

   Both eyes: _____ Acromian process: _____
   Iliac crests: _____ ASIS: _____
   Greater trochanter: _____ Patellae: _____
   Ankle malleoli: _____ Waist angle: _____

   b. Posterior view:

   Earlobes: _____ Spine of the scapula: _____
   Shoulder: _____ Inferior angle of scapula: _____
   Iliac crests: _____ PSIS: _____
   Greater trochanter: _____ Buttocks: _____
   Knee creases: _____ Ankle malleoli: _____
   Spine: _____

   c. Lateral view (see through the line of gravity – Impression): _____
   _____

ii. **Contour and Alignment of Bone and Joints:**
   Impression: _____
   _____

iii. **Size and Contour of Soft Tissue Structure:**

   Soft tissue edema: _____ Joint effusion: _____
   Muscle hypertrophy: _____ Muscle atrophy: _____
   Muscle rupture: _____ Cysts, Rheumatoid nodules: _____
   Ganglion: _____ Gouty tophi: _____
   Impression: _____

iv. **Colour and Texture of Skin:**

   Cyanosis: _____ Pallor: _____
   Erythema (localized, generalized): _____ Yellow skin: _____
   Highly pigmented hairy areas: _____ Open wounds: _____
   Scars: New scar: _____ Old scar: _____
   Thickening, thinning, and hair loss: _____

Palpation

i. Bony Prominence: (Pain, Abnormal Alignment):
   Antr Surface: _____
   Postr Surface: _____
   Lat Surface: (Rt) _____ (Lt) _____

ii. Soft tissue structures:
   Pain: _____ Tenderness (Grade): _____
   Swelling: _____ Spasm: _____
   Nodules: _____ Trigger points: _____
   Fascia tightness: _____ Mobility of soft tissue: _____
   Density and extensibility of soft tissues: _____
   Impression: _____
   _____

iii. Skin:
   Warmth: _____ Density: _____
   Extensibility of skin: _____ Peripheral pulses: _____
   Edema (pitting or non-pitting edema): _____ Grade: _____

Anthropometric Measurements

1. Limb length: (i) True length: (Rt) _____ (Lt) _____
                (ii) Apparent length: (Rt) _____ (Lt) _____
2. Circumference Measurement:
   Upper arm: Rt _____ Lt _____
      Upper :
      Middle:
      Lower :
   Forearm : Rt _____ Lt _____
   Mid-thigh : Rt _____ Lt _____
      Upper :
      Middle:
      Lower :
   Calf : Rt _____ Lt _____
   Chest :
      Upper :
      Middle:
      Lower :

Examination

1. **Assessment of Range of Motion (Attached Annexure-3):**
   (Find the Amount, Quality, Pattern, Pain and Crepitus) AROM, PROM
   Impression: _____
   _____

2. **Assessment of Muscle Strength (Attached Annexure-6):**
   Impression: _____
   _____

3. **Assessment of Muscle Length (Attached Annexure-7):**
   Impression: _____
   _____

4. **Assessment of Sensation** (Attached **Annexure-8**):
   Superficial: _____
   _____
   Deep: _____
   _____

5. **Assessment of Posture** (Attached **Annexure-14**):
   Impression: _____
   _____

6. **Assessment of Gait** (Attached **Annexure-15**):
   Impression: _____
   _____

7. **Assessment of Functional Activity** (Attached **Annexure-16**):
   Impression: _____
   _____

8. **Assessment of Environment** (Attached **Annexure-17**):
   Impression: _____
   _____

9. **External Devices Used:**
   Impression: _____
   _____

10. **Other Systems Examination:**
    Nervous system:
    CVS: DVT/Postural Dysfunction/Edema:
    Respiratory system: Type/Pattern of breathing/Chest expansion/Chest deformities:
    Skin: Pressure sore:
    Bladder/Bowel: Retention/Constipation/Autonomous/Automatic bladder:
    Sexual Function   :
    Physical Diagnosis   :
    Functional Diagnosis :

Professional Diagnosis:
Problem list: _____
_____
_____

Management

Aims : 1.
        2.
        3.
Means : 1.
        2.
        3.

ORTHOSIS POST-PRESCRIPTION ASSESSMENT

LOWER LIMB ORTHOSIS

Standing

- Is the shoe satisfactory and does it fit properly?
- Are the sole and heel of the shoe flat on floor?
- If a shoe insert is used, is there minimal rocking between insert and shoe?

Ankle

- Do the mechanical ankle joints coincide with the anatomical ankle (anatomical ankle joint axis is approximated by a horizontal line between the malleoli at the level of the distal tip of the medial malleolus)?
- Is there adequate clearance between the anatomical ankle and the mechanical ankle joints?
- Does the valgus or varus correction strap control the foot position?

Knee

- Does the mechanical knee joint(s) coincide with the anatomical knee {1.2-1.9 cm} above medial tibial plateau)?
- Is there adequate clearance between the anatomical knee and the mechanical knee joint?
- Is the knee lock sure and easy to operate?

Shells, Bands, Cuffs, and Uprights

- Do the shells, bands, cuffs and uprights conform to the contours of the leg and thigh?
- Is there adequate clearance between the top of the calf shell or band and the head of fibula?
- Is there adequate clearance between the orthosis and the perineum?
- Is the orthosis below the greater trochanter but at least 1 in. higher than the medial shell or upright?
- Are the uprights at the midline of the leg and thigh?
- Do the shells, bands, and cuffs conform to the contours of the leg and thigh?
- Is any flesh roll above the shell or band minimal?
- Are the bottom of the thigh shell or distal thigh band and the top of the calf shell or band equidistance from the knee?
- In a child's orthosis, is there adequate provision for lengthening the orthosis?

Weight-relieving Components

- In a patellar-tendon-bearing brim, is there adequate relief for the head of the fibula?
- With a quadrilateral brim, is the client free from excessive pressure in the anteromedial and medial aspect of the brim?
- With a quadrilateral brim, does the ischial tuberosity rest on the ischial seat?
- With a patellar-tendon-bearing brim, is there adequate reduction in weight bearing through the orthosis?

Hip

- Is the centre of the pelvic joint slightly above and ahead of greater trochanter?
- Is the hip lock secure and easy to operate?
- Does the pelvic band fit the torso accurately?

Sitting

- Can the patient sit comfortably with hips and knees flexed 90°?
- Can patient lean forward to touch the shoes?

Walking

- Is the patient's performance in level walking satisfactory?
- Is the patient's performance on stairs and ramps satisfactory?
- Is the orthosis sufficiently rigid?
- Does the varus or valgus correction strap provide adequate support?
- Does the orthosis operate quietly?
- Does the patient consider the orthosis satisfactory as to comfort, function, and appearance?

Trunk Orthotic Examination

- Is the orthosis as prescribed?
- Can the client don the orthosis easily?

Standing

Pelvic Band

- Does the thoracic band lie flat on the trunk below the scapulae?
- Does the thoracic band lie horizontally on the trunk?

Uprights

- Do the posterior uprights avoid pressure on bony prominences, such as vertebral spines or scapulae?
- Do the lateral uprights extend along the lateral midlines of the trunk?

Abdominal Front

- Is the abdominal front of adequate size?

Cervical Orthosis

- Is the head in the prescribed position?
- Do all rigid components fit properly?

Sitting

- Can the patient sit comfortably with the hips and knee flexed 90°?
- Does the patient consider the orthosis satisfactory as to comfort, function, and appearance?

Orthosis off the Patient

- Is the skin free of abrasions or other discolorations attributable to the orthosis?
- Is the construction satisfactory?
- Do all components function satisfactory?

Prosthesis Prescription Assessment

SUBJECTIVE ASSESSMENT
Demographic Data

Name: _____ Date: _____

Age: _____ Sex: _____

Occupation: _____

Address:

Present: _____ Permanent: _____
        _____   _____
        _____   _____
        _____   _____

Contact No.: Res _____ Off: _____

Referring Doctor: _____ Date of Next Visit: _____

Primary Diagnosis: _____

Case History

Chief Complaints: _____
_____
_____
_____

Past Medical History

Date of Onset: _____

Medical History: _____
_____
_____
_____

i. Previous Medications:

Medicine	Dosage	Frequency
(i) _____	_____	_____
(ii) _____	_____	_____
(iii) _____	_____	_____

ii. Previous Surgeries:

Surgery Name	Date	Complication
(i) _____	_____	_____
(ii) _____	_____	_____
(iii) _____	_____	_____

iii. Previous Diagnostic Test Reports:

*General Medical History (Attached **Annexure-1**):*

Personal History

Family History:

Family Background:

Hereditary complaint:

Occupational History

Related to present illness:

Occupational hazards for illness:

Social History

i. Do you live alone and what type of work do you do in and outside of the home?
ii. How has this problem affected your ability to perform your job?
iii. Do you have to climb stairs to get into your house? Reach the bedroom?

Economic History

1. Onset of Pain:
   a. Sudden: Yes/No, If yes, how? _____
   b. Gradual: Yes/No, If yes, how? _____
   c. Congenital onset: Yes/No, If yes, how? _____
2. Location of Pain: (Through body chart)
   Has the pain change in location: Yes/No, if yes, where _____
   Spread to other areas: Yes/No, if yes, where _____
   Become more focused: Yes/No, if yes, where _____

Prosthesis Prescription Assessment

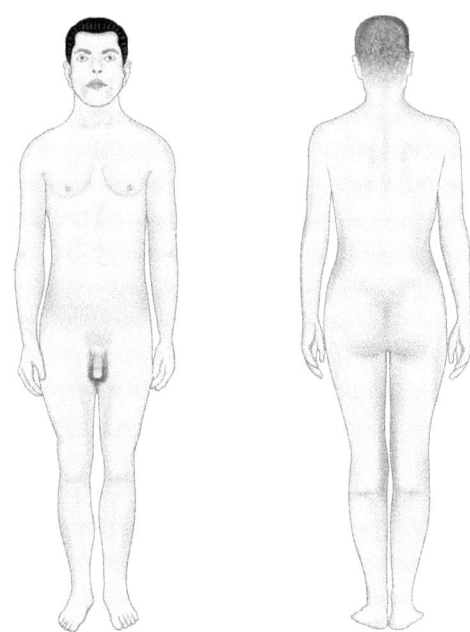

3. Intensity of Pain (Ask the patient to rate his or her pain in this scale):
   Visual Analog Scale:

   No pain   Pain as bad as it could possibly be

OBJECTIVE ASSESSMENT

Mental Status

1. Level of Consciousness :
2. Orientation to
   i. Person :
   ii. Place :
   iii. Time :
3. Vital Signs:

Blood pressure	:	120/80 mmHg
Respiratory rate	:	16–20 /min
Pulse rate	:	72–75
Temperature	:	98.6°F

Observation

General posture: _____
Ability to perform status: _____
Changing the position: _____
Transfer from sitting to standing: _____
Ambulate to the examining room: _____
Built of the Patient: Ectomorphic/Mesomorphic/Endomorphic

Inspection

i. **Postural Alignment:**
   a. Anterior view:

   Both eyes: _____ Acromian process: _____
   Iliac crests: _____ ASIS: _____
   Greater trochanter: _____ Patellae: _____
   Ankle malleoli: _____ Waist angle: _____

   b. Posterior view:

   Earlobes: _____ Spine of the scapula: _____
   Shoulder: _____ Inferior angle of scapula: _____
   Iliac crests: _____ PSIS: _____
   Greater trochanter: _____ Buttocks: _____
   Knee creases: _____ Ankle malleoli: _____
   Spine: _____

   c. Lateral view (see through the line of gravity – Impression): _____
   _____

ii. **Contour and Alignment of Bone and Joints:**
   Impression: _____
   _____

iii. **Size and Contour of Soft Tissue Structure:**

   Soft tissue edema: _____ Joint effusion: _____
   Muscle hypertrophy: _____ Muscle atrophy: _____
   Muscle rupture: _____ Cysts, Rheumatoid nodules: _____
   Ganglion: _____ Gouty tophi: _____
   Impression: _____

iv. **Colour and Texture of Skin:**

   Cyanosis: _____ Pallor: _____
   Erythema (localized, generalized): _____ Yellow skin: _____
   Highly pigmented hairy areas: _____ Open wounds: _____
   Scars: New scar: _____ Old scar: _____
   Thickening, thinning, and hair loss: _____

Palpation

i. **Bony Prominence (Pain, Abnormal Alignment):**
   Antr Surface: _____
   Postr Surface: _____
   Lat Surface: (Rt) _____ (Lt) _____

ii. Soft tissue structures:
   Pain: _____ Tenderness (Grade): _____
   Swelling: _____ Spasm: _____
   Nodules: _____ Trigger points: _____
   Fascia tightness: _____ Mobility of soft tissue: _____
   Density and extensibility of soft tissues: _____
   Impression: _____

iii. Skin:
   Warmth: _____ Density: _____
   Extensibility of skin: _____ Peripheral pulses: _____
   Edema (pitting or non-pitting edema): _____ Grade: _____

Anthropometric Measurements

1. Limb length: (i) True length: (Rt) _____ (Lt) _____
   (ii) Apparent length: (Rt) _____ (Lt) _____
2. Circumference Measurement:
   Upper arm: Rt _____ Lt _____
      Upper :
      Middle:
      Lower :
   Forearm : Rt _____ Lt _____
   Midthigh : Rt _____ Lt _____
      Upper :
      Middle:
      Lower :
   Calf : Rt _____ Lt _____
   Chest :
      Upper :
      Middle:
      Lower :

Examination

1. **Assessment of Range of Motion** (Attached **Annexure-3**):
   (Find the Amount, Quality, Pattern, Pain and Crepitus) AROM, PROM
   Impression: _____

2. **Assessment of Muscle Strength** (Attached **Annexure-6**):
   Impression: _____

3. **Assessment of Muscle Length** (Attached **Annexure-7**):
   Impression: _____

4. **Assessment of Sensation** (Attached **Annexure-8**):
   Superficial: _____
   _____
   Deep: _____
   _____

5. **Assessment of Posture** (Attached **Annexure-14**):
   Impression: _____
   _____

6. **Assessment of Gait** (Attached **Annexure-15**):
   Impression: _____
   _____

7. **Assessment of Functional Activity** (Attached **Annexure-16**):
   Impression: _____
   _____

8. **Assessment of Environment** (Attached **Annexure-17**):
   Impression: _____
   _____

9. **External Devices Used:**
   Impression: _____
   _____

10. **Other Systems Examination:**
    Nervous system:
    CVS: DVT/Postural Dysfunction/Edema:
    Respiratory system: Type/Pattern of breathing/Chest expansion/Chest deformities:
    Skin: Pressure sore:
    Bladder/Bowel: Retention/Constipation/Autonomous/Automatic bladder:
    Sexual Function   :
    Physical Diagnosis   :
    Functional Diagnosis :

Professional Diagnosis:
Problem list: _____
_____
_____

Management

Aims   : 1.
         2.
         3.
Means : 1.
         2.
         3.

CHAPTER 5

Sports Injury Assessment

SUBJECTIVE ASSESSMENT

Demographic Data

Name: _____ Date: _____

Age: _____ Sex: _____

Occupation: _____ Hand dominance: _____

Height: _____ cm   Weight: _____ kg   BMI: _____

Address:

Present: _____ Permanent: _____
_____ _____
_____ _____
_____ _____

Contact No.: Res _____ Off: _____

Referring Doctor: _____ Date of Next Visit: _____

Primary Diagnosis: _____

Case History

Chief Complaints: _____
_____
_____
_____

Past Medical History

Date of Onset: _____

Current Injury history:
- ◆ Stated by the athlete.
    - What is the problem?
    - What hurts?
    - When did the injury occur?
    - What activities or motions are weak or painful?
- ◆ Primary Complaint.
- ◆ Mechanism of Injury
    - How did the injury occur? What did you do? How did you do it?
    - Did you fall? If so, how did you land? WB or NWB?
    - Were you struck by an object or another individual? If so, in what position was the involved body part, and in what speed/direction/intensity/duration was the force?
        - Activity at time of injury?
        - Results of force—twisting, hyperextension/flexion
- ◆ Was a sound heard? By individual or anyone else? Pop, snap, rip?
- ◆ Do you remember a specific incident that initiated or provoked the current problem?
- ◆ Have there been recent changes in running surface, shoes, equipment, techniques, or conditioning modes?
- ◆ Protective Equipment Skill:
    - Protective Equipment:
    - Skill Level:

Medical History Questionnaire

1. What previous care has been sought for the problem?
2. Who else has treated the problem?
3. What tests and treatment did they perform?
4. What have you done to relieve the problem?
5. Has this problem occurred before? If yes, How was it treated or resolved?
  i. Previous Medications:

Medicine	Dosage	Frequency
(i) _____	_____	_____
(ii) _____	_____	_____
(iii) _____	_____	_____

  ii. Previous Surgeries:

Surgery Name	Date	Complication
(i) _____	_____	_____
(ii) _____	_____	_____
(iii) _____	_____	_____

iii. Previous Diagnostic Test Reports:

Surgery Name	Date	Complication
X- Rays: _____	C.T Scan: _____	M.R.I: _____
Bone scan: _____	EMG: _____	Blood test: _____
Myelogram: _____	Biochemical test: _____	Others: _____

Personal History:
Do you use tobacco products? Alcohol? Recreational drugs? If yes,
- Name and Frequency of cigarettes/day _____
- Name and Frequency of Alcohol/day _____
- Name and Frequency of Drugs/day _____

Family History:

Occupational History:

Socio Economic History:

Training History:

Equipment History:

Pain History:
1. Onset of Pain:
   a. Sudden: Yes/No, If yes, how? _____
   b. Gradual: Yes/No, If yes, how? _____
2. Where is pain located now? Where was it located at time of injury? Have athlete point to pain with one finger.
3. Location of Pain (Through body chart):

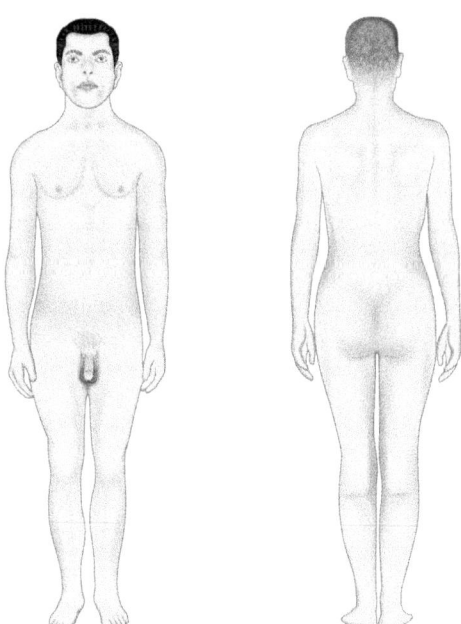

Has the pain change in location: Yes/No, if yes, where _____
Spread to other areas: Yes/No, if yes, where _____
Become more focused: Yes/No, if yes, where _____

4. Intensity of Pain (Ask the patient to rate his or her pain in this scale):
   Visual Analog Scale:

          ⟵⟶

       No pain   Pain as bad as it could possibly be

5. Type of pain (Attached **Annexure-2**):
6. Behavior of symptoms:
   What makes your symptoms increase?
   i. Rest: yes/no, if yes, which position _____
   ii. Activity: yes/no, if yes, which position _____
   iii. Body position: yes/no, if yes, which position _____
   What makes your symptoms decrease?
   i. Rest: yes/no, if yes, which position _____
   ii. Activity: yes/no, if yes, which position _____
   iii. Body position: yes/no, if yes, which position _____
   Behavior of symptom during the last 48 hours:
   Better, worse, staying the same: _____

OBJECTIVE ASSESSMENT

Mental Status

1. Level of Consciousness :
2. Orientation to
   i. Person   :
   ii. Place   :
   iii. Time   :
3. General arousal state :
4. Cognitive state :
5. Communication ability :
6. Vital Signs:
    Blood pressure   :   120/80 mmHg
    Respiratory rate   :   16–20/min
    Pulse rate   :   72–75
    Temperature   :   98.6°F

Observation

General posture: _____
Ability to perform status: _____
Changing the position: _____
Transfer from sitting to standing: _____
Ambulate to the examining room: _____
Built of the patient: Ectomorphic/Mesomorphic/Endomorphic

Inspection

i. **Postural Alignment:**
   a. Anterior view:

Both eyes: _____	Acromion Process: _____
Iliac crests: _____	ASIS: _____
Greater trochanter: _____	Patellae: _____
Ankle Malleoli: _____	Waist angle: _____

   b. Posterior view:

Ear lobes: _____	Spine of the scapula: _____
Shoulder: _____	Inferior angle of scapula: _____
Iliac crests: _____	PSIS: _____
Greater trochanter: _____	Buttocks: _____
Knee creases: _____	Ankle malleoli: _____
Spine: _____	

   c. Lateral view (see through the line of gravity – Impression) _____
   _____
   _____

ii. **Contour and Alignment of Bone and Joints (Fracture and deformity):**
   Impression: _____
   _____

iii. **Size and Contour of Soft Tissue Structure:**

Soft tissue edema: _____	Joint effusion: _____
Muscle hypertrophy: _____	Muscle atrophy: _____
Muscle rupture: _____	Cysts, Rheumatoid nodules: _____
Ganglion: _____	Gouty tophi: _____

   Impression: _____
   _____

Palpation

i. Bony Prominences: (Pain, Abnormal Alignment, Deformity)
   Antr Surface: _____
   Postr Surface: _____
   Lat Surface: (Rt) _____ , (Lt) _____

ii. Soft tissue structures:

Pain: _____	Tenderness (Grade): _____
Swelling: _____	Spasm: _____
Nodules: _____	Trigger points: _____
Fascia tightness: _____	Mobility of soft tissue: _____

   Density and extensibility of soft tissues: _____
   Impression: _____
   _____

iii. Skin:

Warmth: _____	Density: _____
Extensibility of skin: _____	Peripheral pulses: _____
Edema (pitting or non-pitting edema): _____	Grade: _____

Examination

1. **Assessment of Range of Motion** (Attached **Annexure-3**):
   (Find the Amount, Quality, Pattern, Pain and Crepitus) AROM, PROM
   Impression: _____
   _____

2. **Assessment of End Feel** (Attached **Annexure-4**):
   (Feeling which is felt by the therapist as a resistance or a barrier to further motion)
   Impression: _____
   _____

4. **Assessment of Accessory Joint Motion:**
   (If passive ROM is limited or painful assess the accessory joint motion in 1-6 grade)
   Impression: _____
   _____

5. **Assessment of Resisted Isometric Muscle Testing:**
   (Identify the problem in contractile or non-contractile structure – mention the muscle group)
   Impression: _____
   _____

6. **Assessment of Muscle Strength** (Attached **Annexure-6**):
   Impression: _____
   _____

7. **Assessment of Muscle Length** (Attached **Annexure-7**):
   Impression: _____
   _____

8. **Assessment of Hand-held/Isokinetic Dynamometry:**
   Impression: _____
   _____

12. **Assessment of Posture** (Attached **Annexure-14**):
    Impression: _____
    _____

13. **Assessment of Gait** (Attached **Annexure-15**):

Distance walked	Step length difference
Elapsed Time	Cadence
Walking Velocity	Width of Walking Base
Left Stride Length	Left Foot Angle
Right Stride Length	Right Foot Angle
Left Step Length	Right-stride Length to Right L.L Length
Right Step Length	Left-stride Length to Left L.L Length

Impression: _____

14. Assessment of Functional Activity (Attached **Annexure-16**):
Impression: _____

15. Assessment of Environment (Attached **Annexure-17**):
Impression: _____

16. Special Test (Special tests/exams establish degree of injury):
Impression: _____

17. Other Systems Examination:
Nervous system:
CVS: DVT/Postural Dysfunction/Edema:
Respiratory system: Type/Pattern of Breathing/Chest expansion/Chest deformities:
Skin: Pressure sore:
Bladder/Bowel: Retention/Constipation/Autonomous/Automatic bladder:
Sexual function:
Physical Diagnosis :
Functional Diagnosis :

Professional Diagnosis:
Problem list: _____
_____
_____

Management

Short-term Goals

Aims : 1.
2.
3.
4.
5.
Means : 1.
2.
3.
4.
5.

Long-term Goals

Aims : 1.
        2.
        3.
        4.
        5.

Means : 1.
        2.
        3.
        4.
        5.

6
CHAPTER

Sports Fitness Assessment

SUBJECTIVE ASSESSMENT

Demographic Data

Name: _____   Date: _____

Age: _____   Sex: _____

Occupation: _____

Address:

Present: _____   Permanent: _____
        _____   _____
        _____   _____
        _____   _____

Contact No.: Res _____   Off: _____

Referring Doctor: _____

Case History

Chief Complaints: _____
_____
_____
_____

Past Medical History

Questionnaire-1: Physical Activity and Medical History (Yes/No)

1. Has a doctor ever said you have a heart condition and recommended only medically supervised activity?
2. Do you have chest pain brought on by physical activity?
3. Do you tend to lose consciousness or fall over a result of dizziness?
4. Has a doctor ever recommended medication for your blood pressure or a heart condition?
5. Do you have a bone or joint problem that could be aggravated by the proposed physical activity?
6. Are you aware through your own experiences or a doctor's advice, of any other physical reason against your exercising without medical service?
7. Are you over the age of 65 and not accustom to vigorous exercise?

Questionnaire-2: Exercise/Movement Questionnaire (Yes/No)

1. Are you currently involved in an existing exercise program?
2. Are you currently involved in a structured resistance training program?
   ☐ If yes, how long (consistently?) ☐ < 6 months ☐ 6 months to 1 year ☐ > 1 year
3. Are you currently participating in a structured cardiorespiratory program?
   ☐ If yes, _____ days/week, _____ minutes per day, using (mode) _____
4. Other physical activities/interests (including frequency)

Questionnaire-3: Pre-Exercise Questionnaire

1. What is your primary goal?
   ☐ Weight Loss ☐ Muscle Gain ☐ Sport Performance ☐ Improve Health/Daily Activity
2. Specific desires (lbs. weight loss/gain, sport dynamic, aspect of health, etc.)
3. Specific reasons (why? why now? time frame?)
4. Past attempts in obtaining goal (formal/informal programs, successes, challenges, money spent)
5. Goal outcomes (how will you feel when goal is obtained? emotional/physical benefits?)
6. Level of commitment in accomplishing the goal? LOW   HIGH
7. Support/accountability? (Spouse/significant other) _____
8. How much time do you have budgeted? _____ days/weeks; _____ hours/day

Questionnaire-4: Food/Nutrition Questionnaire

1. Typically, how many meals do you eat per day? (circle one)   1 2 3 4 5 6
2. Typically, what time are these meals? _____
3. Typically, how many calories do you consume per day? _____
4. Do you know how many calories you should be eating to reach/support your goal? ☐ YES ☐ NO
   ☐ If YES, how many and how was this determined
5. Are you currently taking a multi-vitamin or any other dietary supplements? ☐ YES ☐ NO
6. How would you describe your diet? ☐ Regular ☐ Lacto-Ovo Vegetarian ☐ Vegan
7. Typically how many meals do you eat outside the home per week? _____
   ☐ Would the majority of these meals be described as: ☐ Fast Food (take-out) ☐ Seated Restaurants
8. How would you rate your eating habits? Very poor/Very good
9. Strengths and Weaknesses? _____

Fitness Evaluation

A. **Assessment of Cardiorespiratory Fitness:**
   a. 1.5 Mile Run Test/1 Mile Walk Test
      Date   :
      Finish time   :
      Fitness category   :
   b. Step Test:
      Date   :
   Recovery Heart Rate Post Exercise (Beats)
      1 – 1.5 min   :
      2 – 2.5 min   :
      3 – 3.5 min   :
      Total   :
      Fitness category   :
   Reason for Termination :

B. **Muscular Strength Assessment:**
   1 R. M Test :
   Muscular Strength = 1 RM (lbs) × 100/Body weight (lbs)

Exercise	1 RM (lbs)	Muscular Strength Score	Fitness Category
Bench Press			
Biceps Curl			
Shoulder Press			
Leg Press			
Squat Test			

C. **Muscular Endurance Assessment:**
   Push-up/modified push–ups:
   Sit ups:
   Number of Push up/Modified push up (1 min) _____
   Fitness Category: _____
   Number of Sit up (1 min) _____
   Fitness Category: _____

D. **Assessment of Flexibility:**
   Sit and reach score (inches): _____
   Fitness Category: _____
   Trunk and Shoulder flexibility score (inches): _____

E. **Body Composition Assessment:**
   1. Skin Fold Test:
      Men:
         Chest _____, Abdominal _____, Thigh _____
         Biceps _____, Triceps _____, Subscapular _____,
         Supra-ilium _____

Women:

    Triceps _____, Supra-ilium _____, Thigh _____

    Subscapular _____, Biceps _____

Sum of three/four skin folds (mm):

Percent body fat :

Fitness Category :

2. Body Mass Index:

   BMI Score   :

   Fitness Score   :

3. Waist to Hip Circumference Ratio:

   Waist Measurement: Hip Measurement: WHR:

   Fitness Category:

4. Girth Measurement: (cm/inches)

      Upper arm   :

      Forearm   :

      Mid-thigh   :

      Calf   :

      Percent Fat :

5. Limb length: (i) True length: (Rt) _____ (Lt) _____

               (ii) Apparent length: (Rt) _____ (Lt) _____

Observation: General Screening

Postural Screen:

Anterior Shoulder Flexibility:

Cervical ROM:

Resisted internal/external rotation:

Full Knee extension/flexion:

Single and Double knee to chest:

Vital Signs:

   Blood pressure   :   120/80 mmHg

   Respiratory rate :   16–20 /min

   Pulse rate   :   72–75

   Temperature   :   98.6°F

Inspection

i. **Postural Alignment:**

   a. Anterior view:

      Both eyes: _____   Acromian Process: _____

      Iliac crests: _____   ASIS: _____

      Greater trochanter: _____   Patellae: _____

      Ankle malleoli: _____   Waist angle: _____

b. Posterior view:

Ear lobes: _____	Spine of the Scapula: _____
Shoulder: _____	Inferior angle of Scapula: _____
Iliac crests: _____	PSIS: _____
Greater Trochanter: _____	Buttocks: _____
Knee creases: _____	Ankle Malleoli: _____
Spine: _____	

c. Lateral view (see through the line of gravity–Impression): _____
_____
_____

ii. **Contour and Alignment of Bone and Joints:**
Impression: _____
_____

Examination

1. **Assessment of Range of Motion** (Attached **Annexure-3**):
   (Find the Amount, Quality, Pattern, Pain and Crepitus) AROM, PROM
   Impression: _____
   _____

2. **Assessment of Muscle Strength** (Attached **Annexure-6**):
   Impression: _____
   _____

3. **Assessment of Nutritional Status** (Attached **Annexure-24**):
   Impression: _____
   _____

4. **Other Systems Examination:**
   Nervous system:
   CVS: DVT/Postural Dysfunction/Edema:
   Respiratory system: Type/Pattern of Breathing/Chest expansion/Chest deformities:
   Skin: Pressure sore:
   Bladder/Bowel: Retention/Constipation/Autonomous/Automatic bladder:
   Sexual function:

Professional Diagnosis:
Problem list: _____
_____
_____

Management

Short-term Goals

Aims : 1.
       2.
       3.
Means : 1.
        2.
        3.

Long-term Goals

Aims : 1.
       2.
       3.
Means : 1.
        2.
        3.

CHAPTER 7

Neurological Assessment

SUBJECTIVE ASSESSMENT

Demographic Data

Name: _____   Date: _____

Age: _____   Sex: _____

Occupation: _____   Handedness: _____

Address:

Present: _____   Permanent: _____
_____   _____
_____   _____
_____   _____

Contact No.: Res _____   Off: _____

Referring Doctor: _____   Date of Next Visit: _____

Primary Diagnosis: _____

Case History

Chief Complaints: _____
_____
_____
_____

Risk Factors: _____

Past Medical History

Date of Onset: _____

Medical History: _____
_____
_____
_____

Medical History Questionnaire

1. What previous care has been sought for the problem?
2. Who else has treated the problem?
3. What tests and treatment did they perform?
4. What have you done to relieve the problem?
5. Has this problem occurred before? If yes, how was it treated or resolved?
    i. Previous Medications:

	Medicine	Dosage	Frequency
(i)	_____	_____	_____
(ii)	_____	_____	_____
(iii)	_____	_____	_____

    ii. Previous Surgeries:

	Surgery Name	Date	Complication
(i)	_____	_____	_____
(ii)	_____	_____	_____
(iii)	_____	_____	_____

    iii. Previous Diagnostic Test Reports:

    X- rays: _____, C.T Scan: _____, M.R.I: _____

    Bone scan: _____, EMG: _____, Blood test: _____

    Myelogram: _____, Biochemical test: _____, Others: _____

*General Medical History (Attached **Annexure-1**):*

Personal History

Do you use tobacco products? Alcohol? Recreational drugs? If yes,
- Name and Frequency of cigarettes/day _____
- Name and Frequency of Alcohol/day _____
- Name and Frequency of Drugs/day _____
    i. What percentage of your normal work activities are you able to perform?
       0% 10% 20% 30% 40% 50% 60% 70% 80% 90% 100%
    ii. What percentage of your normal home activities are you able to perform?
       0% 10% 20% 30% 40% 50% 60% 70% 80% 90% 100%

iii. What percentage of your normal recreational activities are you able to perform?
0% 10% 20% 30% 40% 50% 60% 70% 80% 90% 100%

Family History
- Family Background:
- Hereditary Complaint:

Occupational History
- Related to present illness:
- Occupational hazards for illness:

Social History
i. Do you live alone and what type of work do you do in and outside of the home?
ii. How has this problem affected your ability to perform your job?
iii. Do you have to climb stairs to get into your house? Reach the bedroom?

Economic History
Pain History
1. Onset of Pain:
   a. Sudden: Yes/No, If yes, how? _____
   b. Gradual: Yes/No, If yes, how? _____
   c. Congenital onset: Yes/No, If yes, how? _____
2. Location of Pain: (Through body chart)

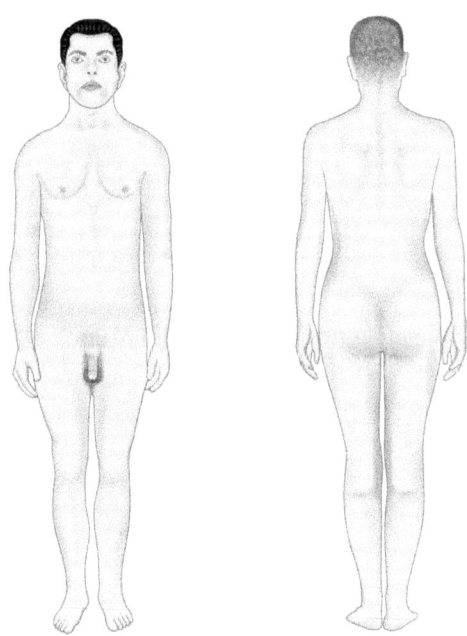

Has the pain change in location: Yes/No, if yes, where _____
Spread to other areas: Yes/No, if yes, where _____
Become more focused: Yes/No, if yes, where _____

3. Intensity of Pain (Ask the patient to rate his or her pain in this scale)
   Visual Analog scale:

   <--->
   No pain   Pain as bad as it could possibly be

4. Type of pain (Attached **Annexure-2**):
5. Behavior of symptoms:
   - What makes your symptoms increase?
   - What makes your symptoms decrease?

OBJECTIVE ASSESSMENT

Higher Mental Status

1. Level of Consciousness:
2. Orientation to
   i. Person :
   ii. Place :
   iii. Time :
3. Memory (Rivermead Behavioural Memory Test)
   i. Immediate :
   ii. Recent :
   iii. Remote :
4. General arousal state :
5. Cognitive state
   1. Fund of Knowledge :
   2. Calculation :
   3. Proverb Interpretation :
6. Perception:
   1. Body scheme/Body image disorders:
      (Unilateral neglect/Anosognosia/Somatoagnosia/Rt-Lt Discrimination)
   2. Spatial relation disorders :
      (Topographic and Vertical orientation/Depth and Distance perception)
   3. Agnosias :
      (Visual/Auditory/Tactile)
   4. Apraxia :
      (Ideamotor/Ideational/Constitutional)
7. Communication ability :
8. Emotional status :
9. Behavior (I – VIII stages) No response (1) to decreased response levels (II & III), confused levels (IV, V, VI), appropriate – automatic, purposeful levels (VII, VIII).
10. Attention state :
    i. Selective attention :
    ii. Sustained attention :
    iii. Alternating attention :
    iv. Divided attention :

11. Speech:
    Type of Speech: Slurred/Nasal/Noisy
    Dysphasia:
    Aphasia: Broca's (receptive)/Wernicke's Aphasia (Expressive)/Global
    Dysarthria:
12. Hearing:
    Normal/Affected
13. Cranial nerve examination (Attached **Annexure-18**):
    Impression: _____
    _____
    _____

14. Vital signs:
    Blood pressure   :   120/80 mmHg
    Respiratory rate :   16–20/min
    Pulse rate   :   72–75
    Temperature   :   98.6° F

Observation

Built of the patient: Ectomorphic/Mesomorphic/Endomorphic
Attitude of limbs: _____
General posture: _____
Ability to perform status: _____
Changing the position: _____
Transfer from sitting to standing: _____
Ambulate to the examining room: _____

Inspection

i. **Postural Alignment:**
   a. Anterior view:
      _____
      _____

   b. Posterior view:
      _____
      _____

   c. Lateral view: _____
      _____

ii. **Contour and Alignment of Bone and Joints:**
    Impression: _____
    _____

iii. **Size and Contour of Soft Tissue Structure:**
     Soft tissue edema: _____   Joint effusion: _____
     Muscle hypertrophy: _____   Muscle atrophy: _____
     Impression: _____
     _____

iv. **Size and Contour of Nails:**
_____
_____
Clubbing (Grade): _____

v. **Colour and Texture of Skin and Tongue:**
Cyanosis: _____ Pallor: _____
Erythema (localized, generalized): _____ Yellow skin: _____
Highly pigmented hairy areas: _____ Open wounds: _____
Scars: New scar: _____ Old scar: _____
Thickening, thinning, and hair loss: _____
_____

Palpation

i. Bony Prominences (Pain, Abnormal Alignment):
   Antr Surface: _____
   Postr Surface: _____
   Lat Surface: (Rt) _____ , (Lt) _____

ii. Soft tissue structures:
   Pain: _____ Tenderness (Grade): _____
   Swelling: _____ Spasm: _____
   Nodules: _____ Trigger points: _____
   Fascia tightness: _____ Mobility of soft tissue: _____
   Density and extensibility of soft tissues: _____

   Tenderness grade: 1: Patient feels pain
                           2: Patient winces
                           3: Patient winces and withdraws
                           4: Patient won't allow to touch
   Impression: _____
   _____

iii. Skin:
   Warmth: _____ Density: _____
   Extensibility of skin: _____ Peripheral pulses: _____
   Edema (pitting or non-pitting edema): _____ Grade: _____

Anthropometric Measurements

1. Limb length: (i) True length: (Rt) _____ (Lt) _____
                (ii) Apparent length: (Rt) _____ (Lt) _____
2. Circumference Measurement:
   Upperarm : Rt _____ Lt _____
   Forearm   : Rt _____ Lt _____
   Mid-thigh : Rt _____ Lt _____
   Calf   : Rt _____ Lt _____
   Chest   : _____

Examination

1. **Assessment of Range of Motion** (Attached **Annexure-3**):
   (Find the Amount, Quality, Pattern, Pain and Crepitus) AROM, PROM
   Impression: _____
   _____

2. **Assessment of Muscle Strength** (Attached **Annexure-6**):
   Impression: _____
   _____

3. **Assessment of Muscle Tone** (Generalized/Local):
   Impression: _____
   _____

4. **Assessment of Muscle Length** (Attached **Annexure-7**):
   Impression: _____
   _____

5. **Assessment of Voluntary Motor Control**:
   Impression: _____
   _____

6. **Assessment of Sensation** (Attached **Annexure-8**):
   Superficial: _____

   Deep: _____
   _____

7. **Assessment of Reflex** (Attached **Annexure-9**):
   Superficial: _____

   Deep: _____
   _____

8. **Assessment of Dermatome/Myotome** (Attached **Annexures-12 and 13**):
   Dermatome: _____

   Myotome: _____
   _____

9. **Assessment of Bladder and Bowel** (Retention/Constipation/Autonomous/Automatic):
   Impression: _____
   _____

10. **Assessment of Special Signs** (Disease specific) **(Annexure-19)**:
    Impression: _____
    _____

11. **Assessment of Involuntary Movements**:
    (Tremor, Chorea, Athetosis, Hemibalismus, Nystagmus)
    Impression: _____
    _____

12. **Assessment of Coordination** (Attached **Annexures 10 and 11**):
    Impression: _____
    _____

13. **Assessment of Balance** (Static and Dynamic Balance):
    Impression: _____
    _____

14. **Assessment of Posture** (Attached **Annexure-14**):
    Impression: _____
    _____

15. **Assessment of Gait** (Attached **Annexure-15**):

Distance walked	Step length difference
Elapsed time	Cadence
Walking velocity	Width of walking base
Left stride length	Left foot angle
Right stride length	Right foot angle
Left step length	Right stride length to Right L.L length
Right step length	Left stride length to Left L.L length

    Impression: _____
    _____

16. **Assessment of Functional Status** (Attached **Annexure-16**):
    Impression: _____

17. **Assessment of Hand Function:** Reaching, Grasping, Releasing
    Impression: _____
    _____

18. **Assessment of Environment** (Attached **Annexure-17**):
    Impression: _____
    _____

19. **External Devices Used:**
    Impression: _____
    _____

20. **Other Systems Examination:**
    - Musculoskeletal System:
      - Pain/Stiffness
      - Fracture
      - Spine mobility/ROM/Deformities
    - CVS: DVT/Postural Dysfunction/Edema:
    - Respiratory System:
      - Type/Pattern of Breathing:
      - Chest expansion: Symmetrical or Asymmetrical:
      - Chest deformities:

- GIT:
- Skin: Pressure sore:
- Sexual function:

Diagnostic tests/Special tests (To confirm Diagnosis):

Impression: _____
_____

Professional Diagnosis:
Physical Diagnosis:
Functional Diagnosis:
(Direct Impairments, Indirect Impairments, Composite Impairments)

Problem list: _____
_____
_____
_____
_____

Management

Short-term Goals

Aims : 1.
       2.
       3.
       4.
       5.
Means : 1.
        2.
        3.
        4.
        5.

Long-term Goals

Aims : 1.
       2.
       3.
       4.
       5.
Means : 1.
        2.
        3.
        4
        5.

CHAPTER 8

Paediatric Assessment

SUBJECTIVE ASSESSMENT

Demographic Data

Name: _____ Date: _____

Chronological Age: _____ Gestational Age: _____ Sex: _____

Parent's Occupation: _____

Date and Time of Birth: _____

Birth Wt of Baby: _____ Present Wt of Baby: _____ Height of Baby: _____

Blood Group: Baby: _____ Mother: _____

Address:

Present: _____ Permanent: _____

Contact No: Res _____ Off: _____

Referring Doctor: _____ Date of Next Visit: _____

Primary Diagnosis: _____

Case History

Chief Complaints: _____

Risk Factors: _____

Past Medical History

Date of Onset: _____

Medical History: _____
_____
_____

Birth History (Attached **Annexure-21**):

Prenatal: _____
_____
_____

Natal: _____
_____
_____

Post-Natal: _____
_____
_____

i. Previous Medications:

	Medicine	Dosage	Frequency
(i)	_____	_____	_____
(ii)	_____	_____	_____
(iii)	_____	_____	_____

ii. Previous Surgeries:

	Surgery Name	Date	Complication
(i)	_____	_____	_____
(ii)	_____	_____	_____
(iii)	_____	_____	_____

iii. Previous Diagnostic Test Reports:

X-rays: _____, C.T Scan: _____, M.R.I: _____

Bone scan: _____, EMG: _____, Blood test: _____

Myelogram: _____, Biochemical test: _____, Others: _____

Family History
Family background:
Hereditary complaint:

Socio Economic History:

OBJECTIVE ASSESSMENT

Observation

- Body Type:
- Behavior:
    - Whether child is alert, irritable or fearful in the session or during particular activities.
    - Child becomes fatigued easily or not during activity.
    - Find out what motivates his action – particular situation, person or special plaything.

    Impression: _____
    _____

- Communication :
    - Observe how the patient interacts with others: By gestures, sounds, hand or finger pointing, speech.

    Impression: _____
    _____

- Attention Span:
    - What catches child's attention?
    - For how much time child's attention is maintained on particular thing?
    - How does parent assist him to maintain attention?
    - What distracts the child?
    - Observe what attracts and what distracts.

    Impression: _____
    _____

- Posture:
    - How much parental support is given?

    Impression: _____
    _____

- Position of the child:
    - Which position does the child prefers to be in?
    - Can child get into that position on his own or with help?
    - With assistance, child makes any effort to go in that position.
    - Symmetry of the child (actively or passively maintained).
    - If involuntary movements present, then in which positions these movements are decreased or increased?

    Impression: _____
    _____

- Postural control and alignment:
    - Postural stabilization and counterpoising in all postures. Proper and equal weight bearing.
    - If the child's centre of gravity appears to be unusually high, resulting in floating legs and poor ability to raise head against gravity.
    - Fear of fall in child due to poor balance.

    Impression: _____
    _____

- Use of limbs and hands:
    - Observe whether the baby is using excessive limb patterns in changing the positions. Observe whether one hand or both hands are used. Type of grasp and release.
    - Attitude of limbs/body parts.

Impression: _____

- ◆ Sensory Aspects:
    - Observe a child's use of vision, hearing, touch, smell, temperature in relevant tasks. Does he enjoy any particular sensation?
    - Whether child enjoys being moved or having position changed?

    Impression: _____

- ◆ Form of Locomotion :
    - How child is carried?
    - Any use of wheelchair or walking aids?
    - Which daily activities motivates child to roll, creep, crawl, bottom shuffle or walk?
    - Involuntary movements.

    Impression: _____

- ◆ Deformities (If Any)
    - Observe any recurring position of the whole child.
    - Any part of the body, which remains in particular position in all Postures.
    - The positional preferences typically seen in spastic cerebral palsies are for mid positions of the body.
    - In the arm, this generally consists of:
        - Shoulder protraction or retraction, adduction and internal rotation, Elbow flexion, Forearm pronation, Wrist and Fingers flexion.
    - In the legs, it includes
        - Hip semi-flexion, internal rotation and adduction, Knee semi-flexion, Ankle plantar flexion, Foot pronation or supination, Toes flexion.
    - Athetoid or dystonic posturing usually incorporates extremes of movement such as total flexion or extension.
    - Windswept deformity of hip: One hip flexed, abducted and externally rotated; other hip flexed, adducted and internally rotated and in danger of posterior dislocation.

    Impression: _____

- ◆ Skin, Hair and Nails:
    - Skin – Key Points
        - Colour: Jaundice, pallor, cyanosis, erythema, ecchymosis
        - Texture and Turgor: Degree of hydration or dehydration
    - Hair: Key Points
        - Course, dry, brittle or depigmented hair may indicate nutrition deficiency or thyroid disorder.
        - Hair tufts on spine or buttocks may indicate spine bifida.
    - Nails: Key Points
    - Inspect for colour, shape, condition, nail biting and infection.
    - Clubbing, Spoon nails, Pitted nails.

    Impression: _____

Anthropometric Measurements

1. Limb length: (i) True length: (Rt) _____ (Lt) _____
   (ii) Apparent length: (Rt) _____ (Lt) _____
2. Circumference Measurement:
   Upperarm : Rt _____ Lt _____
   Forearm : Rt _____ Lt _____
   Mid-thigh : Rt _____ Lt _____
   Calf   : Rt _____ Lt _____
   Chest   : _____
   Head   : _____

Examination

1. **Assessment of Milestones** (Attached **Annexure-22**):
   Impression: _____

2. **Assessment of Social Function:**

Character	Age Range	Achieved Age
Identifies Mother	2–3 Months	
Social Smile	2–3 Months	
Vocalizing in Response to Adult Talk	3–6 Months	
Enjoys Social Play	4–6 Months	
Recognition of Mothers Visuality	4–8 Months	
Displays Stranger Anxiety	4–8 Months	
Distinguish Self from Parents	6–9 Months	

   Impression: _____

3. **Assessment of Range of Motion** (Attached **Annexure-3**):
   Impression: _____

4. **Assessment of Muscle Strength (Paediatric)** (Attached **Annexure-6**):
   Impression: _____

5. **Assessment of Muscle Tone** (Generalized/Local):
   Impression: _____

6. **Assessment of Oromotor Function** (Extraoral and Intraoral):
   Impression: _____

7. **Assessment of Sensation** (Attached **Annexure-8**):
   Superficial: _____

   Deep: _____

Paediatric Assessment

8. **Assessment of Reflex** (Attached **Annexure-9**):
   Superficial: _____

   Deep: _____

9. **Assessment of Bladder and Bowel** (Retention/Constipation/Autonomous/Automatic):
   Impression: _____

10. **Assessment of Special Signs** (Disease specific) (Attached **Annexure-19**):
    Impression: _____

11. **Assessment of Involuntary Movements:**
    (Tremor, Chorea, Athetosis, Hemibalismus, Nystagmus)
    Impression: _____

12. **Assessment of Balance:** (Static and Dynamic Balance) (Attached **Annexures-10 and 11**):
    Impression: _____

13. **Assessment of Posture** (Attached **Annexure-14**):
    Impression: _____

14. **Assessment of Functional Status** (Attached **Annexure-16**):
    Impression: _____

15. **Assessment of Hand Function:** Reaching, Grasping, Releasing
    Impression: _____

16. **Assessment of Gait** (Attached **Annexure-15**):

Distance Walked	Step Length Difference
Elapsed Time	Cadence
Walking Velocity	Width of Walking Base
Left Stride Length	Left Foot Angle
Right Stride Length	Right Foot Angle
Left Step Length	Right Stride Length to Right L.L Length
Right Step Length	Left Stride Length to Left L.L Length

    Impression: _____

17. **External Devices Used:**
    Impression: _____

18. **Other Systems Examination:**
    Musculoskeletal System:
       Pain/Stiffness

       Fracture
       Spine mobility/ROM/Deformities
CVS: DVT/Postural Dysfunction/Edema:
Respiratory system:
       Type/Pattern of Breathing:
       Chest expansion: Symmetrical or Asymmetrical:
       Chest deformities:
GIT:
Skin: Pressure sore:
Sexual function:
Diagnostic tests/Special tests: (To confirm Diagnosis)
Impression: _____

Professional Diagnosis:
Functional Diagnosis:
(Direct Impairments, Indirect Impairments, Composite Impairments)
Problem list: _____

Management

Short-term Goals

Aims : 1.
       2.
       3.
       4.
       5.
Means : 1.
       2.
       3.
       4.
       5.

Long-term Goals

Aims : 1.
       2.
       3.
       4.
       5.
Means : 1.
       2.
       3.
       4
       5.

9 CHAPTER

Cardiac Assessment

SUBJECTIVE ASSESSMENT

Demographic Data

Name: _____ Date: _____

Age: _____ Sex: _____

Occupation: _____

Address:

Present: _____ Permanent: _____
_____ _____
_____ _____
_____ _____

Contact No.: Res _____ Off: _____

Referring Doctor: _____ Date of Next Visit: _____

Primary Diagnosis: _____

Case History

Chief Complaints: _____
_____
_____
_____

Past Medical History

Date of Onset: _____

Medical History:
- History of Present Condition:
  - Onset of the Condition :
  - Duration of the Condition :
  - Progression of the Symptoms :
- Previous Medical History:
  - Previous Attacks :
  - Previous Treatment :
  - Relevant Medical Condition :

Drug History:
(The drugs which might require alterations in physical therapy treatment)
  - Anti-coagulants :
  - Beta-Blockers :
  - Bronchodilators :
- Previous Medications:

Medicine	Dosage	Frequency
(i)		
(ii)		
(iii)		

- Previous Surgeries:

Surgery Name	Date	Complication
(i)		
(ii)		
(iii)		

Previous Diagnostic Test Reports:

X-rays: _____, ECG: _____, P.F.T: _____
ABG: _____, Echo: _____, Blood test: _____
Angiogram: _____, Biochemical test: _____, Others: _____

General Medical History (Attached Annexure-1):

Personal History

Do you use tobacco products? Alcohol? Recreational drugs? If yes,
- Name and Frequency of Cigarettes/day _____
- Name and Frequency of Alcohol/day _____
- Name and Frequency of Drugs/day _____

Hobbies/Lifestyle: _____
Diet: _____

Family History
- Family Background :
- Hereditary Complaint :

Occupational History
- Related to present illness :
- Occupational hazards :

Social History

OBJECTIVE ASSESSMENT

1. **Assessment of Pain**
- Pericardial pain: No tenderness only deep inspiration causes sharp pain.
- Skeletal pain: Rib # (Localized, Movement aggravates Pain, Tenderness)
- Muscle pain: Due to chronic cough, Pain varies If spasm + ve.
- Neuralgic pain: Herpes zoster, Intercostals nerves affected
- Angina (Strangulation): Stable/Unstable/M.I
- Pain at incision site: Any thoracic surgery.
    i. Character of Pain :
    ii. Duration of Pain :
    iii. Location of Pain :
    iv. Behavior of Pain :
    If Angina present, note down Angina Grade (Use NYHS Scale)
    i. Type : Stable/Unstable/Variant
    ii. Severity :
    iii. Duration :
    Associated Symptoms (Specify)
2. **Assessment of Dyspnoea:**
    (I – Strenuous activity, II – Ordinary activity, III – < ordinary activity, IV – At rest)
    Dyspnoea Grade :

On Observation

A. Level of Consciousness: (Alert, Coma, Confused, Paralysed)
B. Orientation to: Person/Place/Time
C. Built of the Patient: Ectomorphic/Mesomorphic/Endomorphic
D. Posture (Thoracotomy – Scoliosis, Median Sternotomy – Kyphosis):
E. Face and Neck;
   a. General;
      i. Colour, temperature, sweat.
      ii. Malar flush (cheeks – mitral stenosis).

b. Eyes;
      i. Corneal arcus (cholesterol crystals in periphery of cornea).
      ii. Xanthelasma (hyperlipidaemia).
      iii. Anaemia (bottom eyelid).
      iv. Jaundice (sclera).
   c. Tongue;
      i. Central cyanosis (under tongue).
      ii. Dentition (infective endocarditis).
   d. Neck: Distension of neck veins – In RHF.
F. Chest: Chest wall deformities, Incision over chest, Drains/Bandage
   Symmetry of Movement – Paradoxical or Not.
   Pattern of Breathing – Rate, Depth, Rhythm.
G. Respiration:
   i. Rate of Respiration   :
   ii. Pattern of Respiration   :
H. Extremity Evaluation:
   1. Clubbing: (In fingers and Toes)
      a. Stage   :
      b. Idiopathic reason :
      c. Hypoxemia   :
   2. Cyanosis:
      a. Peripheral   :
      b. Central   :
   3. Anemia   :
   4. Capillary refill time :
   5. Edema   :
   6. Tremor   :
   7. Skin changes   :
   8. Soft tissue changes :
   9. Joint deformities   :
   10. External appliances (Head to Toe):
   (Endotracheal Tube, Ventilator (rate and mode setting), Mask, Catheters (venous and urinary), Crepe bandage and stockings, Ryle's tube.)
   Impression: _____
   _____
   _____

On Palpation

1. Tracheal shift:
2. Tenderness (From distal site to painful site):
3. Chest expansion
   Axillary level:

Nipple level   :
   Xiphisternal level   :
4. Accessory muscle palpation:
   SCM   :
   Scalene   :
5. Pulse   :
6. Edema   :
7. Capillary filling (Apex beat, Heaves, Thrills):
8. Bony prominences :
9. Soft tissue structures:
10. Skin and Nails:
    Impression: _____
    _____
    _____
    _____
    _____

Examination of the Radial Pulse

a. Rate and rhythm (normal rate is 60-100 bpm. Irregularly irregular suggests AF. Regularly irregular suggests second degree heart block).
b. Radio-radial delay (delay of L radial compared to R–coarctation of the aorta proximal to the L subclavian artery).
c. Radio-femoral delay (coarctation of the aorta).
d. Collapsing pulse (water-hammer – aortic regurgitation, patent ductus arteriosum).
   Impression: _____
   _____

Examination of the Brachial Artery

a. Both sitting and standing (>15/20 mm Hg difference – orthostatic/postural hypotension).
b. In right and left arm (>10 mm Hg difference is a sign of aortic dissection or coarctation of the aorta. Make a note to always use the arm that gives the higher reading).
   Impression: _____
   _____

Examination of the Carotid Artery

a. Assess character and volume.
b. Low volume, plateau pulse and slow rising (aortic stenosis).
c. Rapid upstroke and down stroke (aortic regurgitation).
d. Auscultate for bruits, moving the diaphragm up the artery (atherosclerosis, aortic stenosis).
   Impression: _____
   _____

Examination of JVP (Jugular Venous Pressure)

a. Measure vertical height (cm) from sternal angle to top of jugular venous pulsation. Norm. is 7 mm Hg.
b. If difficulty finding JVP, apply abdominal pressure for 5–10 secs (hepatojugular reflux) to amplify its presence.
c. Can be distinguished from the carotid pulse commonly by its double peaked wave form (right atrial contraction and atrial filling during ventricular systole) and also by palpation.
d. Elevated JVP in R-sided HF, PE, pericardial effusion/constriction and sup. vena caval obstruction. Altered wave pulsation in – AF, tricuspid stenosis/regurgitation, complete heart block.
Impression: _____

On Percussion:
- Normal – Resonant,
- Air-filled areas – Hyperresonant,
- Consolidated area – Hyporesonant
- Cardiac dullness - Dull

Response:

On Auscultation
- Lung sounds :
- Added sounds:
- Heart sounds :
- Murmur :

Regions: Aortic, Pulmonary, Tricuspid, Mitral.

Assessment of Posture (Attached Annexure-14):
Impression: _____

Assessment of Function (Attached Annexure-16):
Impression: _____

Assessment of Environment (Attached Annexure-17):
Impression: _____

Other Systems Examination

- Musculoskeletal system :
- Nervous system :
- Respiratory system :
- GIT :
- Skin: Pressure sore :
- Bladder/Bowel :
- Retention/Constipation/Autonomous/Automatic bladder :
- Sexual function :

Diagnostic tests/Special tests (To confirm Diagnosis):
Impression: _____
_____

Professional Diagnosis:
Impression: _____
_____

Problem list: _____
_____
_____

Management

Short-term Goals

Aims : 1.
        2.
        3.
        4.
        5.

Means : 1.
         2.
         3.
         4.
         5.

Long-term Goals

Aims : 1.
        2.
        3.
        4.
        5.

Means : 1.
         2.
         3.
         4
         5.

10
CHAPTER

Peripheral Vascular Disease Assessment

SUBJECTIVE ASSESSMENT

Demographic Data

Name: _____ Date: _____

Age: _____ Sex: _____

Occupation: _____

Height: _____ cm Weight: _____ kg BMI: _____

Address:

Present: _____ Permanent: _____
_____ _____
_____ _____
_____ _____

Contact No.: Res _____ Off: _____

Referring Doctor: _____ Date of Next Visit: _____

Primary Diagnosis: _____

Case History

Chief Complaints: _____
_____
_____
_____

Past Medical History

Date of Onset: _____

Medical History:
- ♦ History of Present Condition:
  - Onset of the Condition :
  - Duration of the Condition :
  - Progression of the Symptoms :
- ♦ Previous Medical History:
  - Previous Attacks :
  - Previous Treatment :
  - Relevant Medical Condition :

Drug History:
(The drugs which might require alterations in physical therapy treatment)
- ♦ Associated Problems:
- ♦ Previous Medications:

Medicine	Dosage	Frequency
(i) _____	_____	_____
(ii) _____	_____	_____
(iii) _____	_____	_____

- ♦ Previous Surgeries:

Surgery Name	Date	Complication
(i) _____	_____	_____
(ii) _____	_____	_____
(iii) _____	_____	_____

- ♦ Previous Diagnostic Test Reports:

X-rays: _____, ECG: _____, P.F.T: _____
ABG: _____, Echo: _____, Blood test: _____
Angiogram: _____, Biochemical test: _____, Others: _____

General Medical History (Attached **Annexure-1**):

Personal History:
Do you use tobacco products? Alcohol? Recreational drugs? If yes,
- ♦ Name and Frequency of Cigarettes/day _____
- ♦ Name and Frequency of Alcohol/day _____
- ♦ Name and Frequency of Drugs/day _____

Hobbies/Lifestyle: _____
Diet: _____

Family History:
- Family Background :
- Hereditary Complaint :

Occupational History:
- Related to Present Illness :
- Occupational Hazards :

Social History:

Risk Factor Assessment:

Norton Risk Assessment Scale

Impression: _____

Gosnell Scale – Pressure Sore Risk Assessment

Impression: _____

Braden Scale for Predicting Pressure Sore Risk

Impression: _____

Pain Assessment (PVD):

Intermittent claudication and Rest pain- rate by Walking Impairment Questionnaire

Impression: _____

i. Character of Pain :
ii. Duration of Pain :
iii. Location of Pain :
iv. Behavior of Pain :

Aggravating factors :

Relieving factors :

Different Questionnaires :

Peripheral Vascular Diseases Questionnaire: _____

Peripheral Arterial Diseases Questionnaire: _____

OBJECTIVE ASSESSMENT

Observation

A. Level of Consciousness: (Alert, Coma, Confused, Paralysed)
B. Built of the Patient: (Ectomorphic/Mesomorphic/Endomorphic)
C. Posture:
D. Head and Face Evaluation:
   Facial distress: Cyanotic changes:
E. Neck/Chest:
F. Extremity Evaluation:
   1. Clubbing (In Fingers and Toes):
      a. Stages:
      b. Idiopathic reason:
      c. Hypoxemia:

2. Cyanosis:
    a. Peripheral (PVD, Nicotine stains)
    b. Central (Mucosa)
3. Edema (Dependent/PVD)
   Grading of lymphedema: _____
4. Tremor (Over use of Bronchodilators)
5. Skin Changes (Colour of skin, hair changes)
6. Wound Examination-Size and depth and staging of pressure ulcer
7. External Appliances (Head to Toe):
    i. Endotracheal Tube:
    ii. Ventilator (Rate and mode setting)
    iii. Mask:
    iv. Catheters (Venous and urinary):
    v. Crepe Bandage and Stockings:
    vi. Ryle's tube:
G. Vital Signs:
   Blood pressure   :   120/80 mm Hg
   Respiratory rate :   16–20/min
   Pulse rate   :   72–75

(The cervical and supraclavicular fossae areas, the femoral arteries at the groin level, popliteal, dorsalis pedis, and posterior tibial sites, periumbilical region and the iliac regions.)

   Grade of pulse   :
   Temperature   : 98.6° F
   Ankle Brachial Indices :

Inspection

i. Postural Alignment:
   Impression: _____
   _____

ii. Size and Contour of Nails:
   _____
   _____

iii. Colour and Texture of Skin and Tongue:
   Cyanosis: _____   Pallor: _____
   Erythema (localized, generalized): _____   Yellow skin: _____
   Highly pigmented hairy areas: _____   Open wounds: _____
   Scars: New scar: _____   Old scar: _____
   Thickening, thinning, and hair loss: _____
   _____

Palpation

i. Bone/Soft tissue structures:
   Impression: _____
   _____

ii. Skin:
   Warmth: _____ Density: _____
   Extensibility of skin: _____ Peripheral pulses: _____
   Edema (Pitting or non-pitting edema): _____ Grade: _____

Anthropometric Measurements

Circumference Measurements
Upper arm:
Forearm   :
Mid-thigh :
Calf   :
Chest   :
Volumetric measurement by special container that contain water: _____

Examination

1. **Examination of the hands:**
   a. Peripheral cyanosis (Colour, temperature and sweat).
   b. Clubbing (Cyanotic congenital heart disease, infective endocarditis, atrial myxoma).
   c. Capillary refill time (Press for 5 secs).
   d. Anaemia (Check palmar creases for colour).
2. **Examination of the radial pulse:**
   a. Rate and rhythm (Norm. rate is 60–100 bpm. Irregularly irregular suggests AF. Regularly irregular suggests second degree heart block).
   b. Radio-radial delay (Delay of L radial compared to R – coarctation of the aorta proximal to the L subclavian artery).
   c. Radio-femoral delay (Coarctation of the aorta).
   d. Collapsing pulse (Water-hammer – aortic regurgitation, patent ductus arteriosus).
3. **Examination of the brachial artery:**
   a. Blood pressure:
   i. Both sitting and standing (>15/20 mm Hg difference – orthostatic/postural hypotension).
   ii. In right and left arm (>10 mm Hg difference is a sign of aortic dissection or coarctation of the aorta. Make a note to always use the arm that gives the higher reading).
4. **Examination of the carotid artery:**
   a. Assess character and volume.
   b. Low volume, plateau pulse and slow rising (aortic stenosis).
   c. Rapid upstroke and down stroke (aortic regurgitation).
   d. Auscultate for bruits, moving the diaphragm up the artery (atherosclerosis, aortic stenosis).
5. **Examination of JVP (jugular venous pressure):**
   a. Measure vertical height (cm) from sternal angle to top of jugular venous pulsation. Norm. is 7 mm Hg. No more than 4 cm above the sternal angle.

b. If difficulty finding JVP, apply abdominal pressure for 5–10 secs (hepatojugular reflux) to amplify its presence.
c. Can be distinguished from the carotid pulse commonly by its double peaked waveform (right atrial contraction and atrial filling during ventricular systole) and also by palpation.
d. Elevated JVP in R-sided HF, PE, pericardial effusion/constriction and sup. vena caval obstruction. Altered wave pulsation in – AF, tricuspid stenosis/regurgitation, complete heart block. (NB. Can also be elevated in pregnancy, fluid overload hypertension, Kussmaul's sign – cardiac tamponade)

Special Tests

1. **Arterial Inefficiency**
   Rubor of dependency :
   Air plethysmography (APG) :
   Transcutaneous oxygen pressure ($TcPO_2$) measurement :
   Skin perfusion pressure (SPP) measurement :
   Arteriography :
2. **Venous Inefficiency**
   Venous filling time :
   Percussion test :
   Air plethysmography (APG) :
   Venography/ Phlebography :
3. **DVT**
   Homan's sign :
   Cuff test :
   Trendelenberg test :
4. **Lymphatic Disorder**
   Stemmer's test :
   Lymphoscintigraphy :
   Bioimpedance analysis :
   Impression: _____
   _____

Assessment of Sensation (Attached **Annexure-8**):
Superficial: _____
_____

Deep: _____

Assessment of Posture (Attached **Annexure-14**):
Impression: _____

Assessment of Gait (Attached **Annexure-15**):
Impression: _____

Assessment of Functional Activity (Attached **Annexure-16**):
Impression: _____

Assessment of Environment (Attached **Annexure-17**):
Impression: _____
_____

Other Systems Examination:
- Musculoskeletal system:
- Nervous system:
- Automatic:
- CVS:
- Respiratory system:
- GIT:
- Skin: Pressure sore:
- Bladder/Bowel:
    - Retention:
    - Constipation:
    - Autonomous/Automatic bladder:
- Sexual function:

Diagnostic tests/Special tests (To confirm diagnosis):
I. Investigation
Impression: _____
_____

Professional Diagnosis:

Problem list: _____
_____
_____

Management

Short-term Goals

Aims : 1.
        2.
        3.
        4.
        5.

Means : 1.
        2.
        3.
        4.
        5.

Long-term Goals

Aims : 1.
        2.
        3.
        4.
        5.

Means : 1.
        2.
        3.
        4
        5.

Respiratory Assessment

SUBJECTIVE ASSESSMENT

Demographic Data

Name: _____   Date: _____

Age: _____   Sex: _____

Occupation: _____

Height: _____ cm   Weight: _____ kg   BMI: _____

Address:

Present: _____   Permanent: _____
_____   _____
_____   _____
_____   _____

Contact No.: Res _____   Off: _____

Referring Doctor: _____   Date of Next Visit: _____

Primary Diagnosis: _____

Case History

Chief Complaints: _____
_____
_____
_____

Past Medical History

Date of Onset: _____

Medical History:
- History of Present Condition:
  - Onset of the Condition   :
  - Duration of the Condition :
  - Progression of the Symptoms :
- Previous Medical History:
  - Previous Attacks   :
  - Previous Treatment   :
  - Relevant Medical Condition :

Drug History:
(The drugs which might require alterations in physical therapy treatment)
  - Anticoagulants   :
  - β-Blockers   :
  - Bronchodilators :
- Associated problems :
- Previous Medications :

Medicine	Dosage	Frequency
(i) _____	_____	_____
(ii) _____	_____	_____
(iii) _____	_____	_____

- Previous Surgeries:

Surgery Name	Date	Complication
(i) _____	_____	_____
(ii) _____	_____	_____
(iii) _____	_____	_____

- Previous Diagnostic Test Reports:

X- rays: _____, ECG: _____, P.F.T: _____
ABG: _____, Echo: _____, Blood test: _____
Angiogram: _____, Biochemical test: _____, Others: _____

*General Medical History (Attached **Annexure-1**):*

Personal History

Do you use tobacco products? Alcohol? Recreational drugs? If yes,
- Name and Frequency of Cigarettes/day _____
- Name and Frequency of Alcohol/day _____
- Name and Frequency of Drugs/day _____

Hobbies/Lifestyle: _____
Diet: _____

Family History
- Family Background   :
- Hereditary Complaint :

Occupational History
- Related to present illness :
- Occupational hazards   :

Social History:

OBJECTIVE ASSESSMENT

On Observation

A. Level of Consciousness: (Alert, Coma, Confused, Paralysed)
B. Orientation to: Person/ Place/ Time
C. Built of the Patient:
   - Obese with signs of lung obstruction – COPD Type A (Blue Blotters)
   - Thin with signs of lung obstruction – COPD Type B (Pink Buffers)
   - Thin – Chronic infections, T.B, Supportive lesions, Malnutrition, CHD
D. Posture:
   - Mention the Level:
     - Thorocotomy – Scoliosis
     - Median Sternotomy – Kyphosis
E. Head and Face Evaluation:
   - Facial distress:
   - Cyanotic changes:
F. Neck:
   - Use of accessory muscles – Demand increase
   (Seen in Emphysema and Asthma – Lead to TOS – Because of continuous use of scalene muscles)
   Distension of neck veins – In RHF (Distension of neck veins, Pedal edema, Hepatosplenomegaly)
G. Chest:
   - Unmoving Chest:
     a. Chest wall deformities – Barrel chest
                               – Pigeon chest
                               – Funnel chest
     b. Incision over chest   – Extend of incision
                               – Mention drains/Bandages
     c. Any ICD: Upper   – Pneumothorax
                               – Lower–Effusion

- Moving Chest:
    a. Symmetry of movement – Paradoxical or Not
    b. Pattern of Breathing – Rate, Depth, Rhythm
        Euphoria – Normal pattern, Tachypnoea – Increase rate, Bradypnoea – Decrease rate, Hyperpnoea – Increase depth, shallow breathing – in surgery.
    c. Inspiration / Expiration Ratio: 1:2 (or) 1:3
    d. Expansion: Chest wall expansion due to spinal cord injury.
- **Extremity Evaluation:**
    1. Clubbing: (In fingers and toes)
        a. Stages:
        b. Idiopathic reason:
        c. Hypoxemia:
    2. Cyanosis:
        a. Peripheral - (PVD, Nicotine stains)
        b. Central - (Mucosa)
    3. Edema: (Dependent/PVD)
    4. Tremor: (Over use of Bronchodilators)
    5. Skin Changes:
    6. Joint Deformities:
    7. External Appliances (Head to Toe):
        i. Endotracheal Tube:
        ii. Ventilator: (rate and mode setting)
        iii. Mask:
        iv. Catheters: (venous and urinary)
        v. Crepe bandage and Stockings:
    8. Ryle's tube:

H. Vital Signs:
  - Blood pressure   : 120/80 mm Hg
  - Respiratory rate   : 16-20 /min
  - Pulse rate   : 72-75
  - Temperature   : 98.6° F
  - Built of the Patient : Ectomorphic/Mesomorphic/Endomorphic
  - Respiratory Distress   :
  - Type of Respiration   : Spontaneous/Artificial
  - Supplemental O_2 :
  - Shape:
    (Kyphosis/Kyphoscoliosis/Pectus Excavatum/Pectus Carinatum/Hyperinflation)
  - Respiration:
    i. Rate of Respiration   :
    ii. Pattern of Respiration :
  - Intercostal retraction   :

On Examination

1. **Pain Assessment:**
   - Pleuritic pain - No tenderness only deep inspiration causes sharp pain.
   - Skeletal pain - Rib # (Localized, Movement aggravates pain, Tenderness)
   - Muscle pain - Due to chronic cough, Pain varies If spasm + ve.
   - Neuralgic pain - Herpes zoster, Intercostals nerves affected
   - Angina (Strangulation) - Unstable Angina, Angina – Stable/Unstable/M.I
   - Pain at incision site – Any thoracic surgery.
     - i. Character of Pain   :
     - ii. Duration of Pain   :
     - iii. Location of Pain   :
     - iv. Behavior of Pain   :

   If Angina present, note down Angina Grade (Use NYHS Scale)
   - i. Type: Stable/Unstable/Variant
   - ii. Severity   :
   - iii. Duration   :

   Associated Symptoms (Specify)

2. **Breathlessness:**
   (I – Strenuous activity, II – Ordinary activity, III – < ordinary activity, IV – At rest - NYHA)
   Dyspnoea Grade   :

3. **Cough:**
   - Effectiveness of Cough   :
   - Variations in Cough   :
   - Productive/Non-productive :

   Nocturnal Cough – Common in strokes, interstitial lung diseases.
   Productive Cough – Chronic bronchitis, Asthma
   Severe Productive Cough – Early morning bronchiectasis

4. **Sputum:**
   i. Colour: Green – Pseudomonas, Black – Smokers, Cold mines, Pink frothy – Pulmonary edema, Bloody – Hemoptysis, Carcinoma, T.B, Bronchiectasis, CHD
   ii. Quantity: Normal – 100 ml/day
   iii. Quality: M1 – Mucoid, M2 – Suspicious about Purulence, M3 – 1/3 Purulent, M4 – 2/3 Purulent, M5 – ¾ Purulent
   iv. Consistency: Mucoid, Purulent, Mucopurulent, Tenacious and Thick
   v. Odor: Foul smelling infection, Bronchiectasis

4. **Wheeze:**
   - Diurnal variations   :
   - Positional variations   :
   - Aggravating factors   :

5. **Special Examination:**
   i. **Examination of the hands:**
      a. Peripheral cyanosis (colour, temperature and sweat).
      b. Clubbing (cyanotic congenital heart disease, infective endocarditis, atrial myxoma).

c. Splinter haemorrhages (5+ on one hand is significant. Check occupation. May suggest infective endocarditis).
d. Capillary refill time (press for 5 secs).
e. Tendon xanthomata (fatty deposits in tendons - hyperlipidaemia).
f. Anaemia (check palmar creases for colour).
g. Osler's nodes (painful swellings on tips of fingers, suggestive of infective endocarditis).
h. Janeaway lesions (small red pimples on pulps of hands. Differentiated from Osler's by; being painless and blanching on compression).
i. Tar stains (white fatty deposits on palms).
j. Rheumatoid signs (ulnar deviation, swan neck and suggestive of multisystem disease).

ii. **Examination of the radial pulse:**
   a. Rate and rhythm (norm. rate is 60–100 bpm. Irregularly irregular suggests AF. Regularly irregular suggests second degree heart block).
   b. Radio-radial delay (delay of L radial compared to R – coarctation of the aorta proximal to the L subclavian artery).
   c. Radio-femoral delay (coarctation of the aorta).
   d. Collapsing pulse (water-hammer – aortic regurgitation, patent ductus arteriosus).

iii. **Examination of the brachial artery:**
   a. **blood pressure**
      i. Both sitting and standing (>15/20 mm Hg difference – orthostatic / postural hypotension).
      ii. In right and left arm (>10 mm Hg difference is a sign of aortic dissection or coarctation of the aorta. Make a note to always use the arm that gives the higher reading).

iv. **Examination of the carotid artery:**
   a. Assess character and volume.
   b. Low volume, plateau pulse and slow rising (aortic stenosis).
   c. Rapid upstroke and down stroke (aortic regurgitation).
   d. Auscultate for bruits, moving the diaphragm up the artery (atherosclerosis, aortic stenosis).

v. **Examination of JVP (jugular venous pressure):**
   a. Measure vertical height (cm) from sternal angle to top of jugular venous pulsation. Norm. is 7 mm Hg, –no more than 4 cm above s.a.
   b. If difficulty finding JVP, apply abdominal pressure for 5-10 secs (hepatojugular reflux) to amplify its presence.
   c. Can be distinguished from the carotid pulse commonly by its double peaked wave form (right atrial contraction and atrial filling during ventricular systole) and also by palpation.
   d. Elevated JVP in R-sided HF, PE, pericardial effusion/constriction and sup. vena caval obstruction. Altered wave pulsation in – AF, tricuspid stenosis/regurgitation, complete heart block. (NB. Can also be elevated in pregnancy, fluid overload, hypertension, Kussmaul's sign – cardiac tamponade)

vi. **Examination of the face:**
   a. **General**
      i. Colour, temperature, sweat.
      ii. Malar flush (cheeks – mitral stenosis).
   b. **Eyes**
      i. Corneal arcus (cholesterol crystals in periphery of cornea. In young associated with hypercholesterolaemia, association weakens with age –arcus senilis).
      ii. Xanthelasma (hyperlipidaemia).

iii. Anaemia (bottom eyelid).

iv. Jaundice (sclera).

c. **Tongue;**

i. Central cyanosis (under tongue).

ii. Dentition (infective endocarditis).

vii. **Examine the chest (NB. Dextrocardia possible!)**

On Palpation

Trachea:

(A normal trachea may be shifted slightly to the right)

Surgical Emphysema:

1. Tracheal shift (with three fingers):

   (Palpate with middle finger)
   - Same side shift (Atelactasis, Lobectomy, Pneumonectomy), Opposite side shift (Pneumothorax, Pleural effusion, Haemothorax, Haemopneumothorax)

2. Tenderness:

   (From distal site to painful site)

3. Chest Expansion:
   - Axillary level   :
   - Nipple level   :
   - Xiphisternal level :

4. Accessory muscle palpation:
   - SCM   :
   - Scalene :

5. Tactile fremitus:

   (Ask the patient in sitting position, and ask him to say something.)
   - Consolidation: (sound felt distantly)
   - Pneumothorax/effusion: (Decreased)

6. Movement of Diaphragm:

   (Thumps under the xiphisternum and ask the patient to inspire and expire and feel the movement of Diaphragm)

7. Pulse:

8. Edema:

9. Capillary filling:

   i. Feel for apex beat (5th intercostals space, mid-clavicular line, not position and character).

   ii. Feel for heaves (flat of hand over sternum –R-HF, mitral stenosis, pulmonary hypertension).

   iii. Feel for thrills (side of hand horizontal under left clavicle –aortic/ pulmonary stenosis).

On Percussion

- On intercostal suction always compare with other side.
  - Normal – Resonant
  - Air filled areas – Hyper-resonant

- Consolidated area – Hyporesonant – dull
- Cardiac dullness 3rd to 5th and 4th to 6th
- Normal Response:
  - Anteriorly :   till 6th rib
  - Laterally :   till 8th rib
  - Posteriorly: till 10th rib

  (Don't percuss over the scapula)
- Hyper-Resonant   :
- Normal   :
- Dull   :
- Stony Dull   :

On Auscultation

Lung sounds:
1. Normal sounds:
   a. Tracheal sounds:
      - High pitched sounds
      - Only over trachea
      - Inspiration and Expiration with a pause.
   b. Bronchial sounds:
      - Adjacent to manubrium
      - Not as loud as trachea
      - If this heard over periphery – consolidation
      - Pause between Inspiration and Expiration
   c. Bronchovesicular:
      - Moderate pitch and intensity
      - Area: Angle of Lewis, between scapula
   d. Vesicular (Breath sounds)
      - Very soft and muffled breeze through leaves
      - Heard due to Turbulence
      - Pause decreases
      - Heard in all Peripheral areas
      - Air is not entering from central to periphery (Pneumothorax, Effusion)
      - Hyperinflated lung (Asthma)
      - Any Obstruction – complete absence
2. Voice sounds: (Same as tactile fremitus)
   - Bronchophony – 99,123, etc
   - Egophony – E to A (Say E, E – hear as 'A')
   - Whispering pectoriloquy:
     - Whispering only
     - Normally nothing is heard
     - In consolidation – Distinct sound heard

3. Added sounds:
   a. Wheeze/Bronchi:
      - Air coming through the obstructed pathway
      - Musical and Rhythmic
      - Bronchospasm (Asthma)
      - Common in Expiration
      - Heard both during inspiration and expiration: Chronic Bronchitis
   b. Crepitations/Rales:
      - Due to Secretions
      - Opening of closed Airways
      - Heard clearly during deep inspiration

- Lung sounds   :
- Added sounds   :
- Heart sounds   :
    i. First screen; whilst palpating CA, listen in all 4 regions with both bell and diaphragm, noting no. of heart sounds (s3 norm. in most cases, s4 always abnormal.) and any additional sounds.
    ii. 4 Regions – Aortic (2nd ICS, RSE), Pulmonary (2nd ICS, LSE), Tricuspid (4th ICS, LSE, pt leaning forward, breath held in exp.),
        Mitral (4th ICS, MCL). also Mitral regurgitation. (pt on L side, listen medial to axillary line), apex (5th ICS, MCL).
    iii. If suspected murmur
    iv. Describe as:
        1. Systolic/Diastolic.
        2. Ejection/Pansystolic.
        3. High/Low.
        4. Grade 1-4.
        5. Influence of respiration (L sided murmurs are increased on expiration and R sided decreased).
        6. Radiation (carotids in aortic stenosis, axilla in mitral regurg.).
        7. Influence of rolling on L side (mitral stenosis at the apex).
        8. On sitting forward in expiration (aortic regurg. and stenosis).

On Inspection

i. Postural Alignment:
Impression: _____
_____

ii. Size and Contour of Nails:
_____
_____

iii. Colour and Texture of Skin and Tongue:
Cyanosis: _____ Pallor: _____
Erythema (localized, generalized): _____ Yellow skin: _____
Highly pigmented hairy areas: _____ Open wounds: _____

Scars: New scar: _____ Old scar: _____

Thickening, thinning, and hair loss: _____

_____

Assessment of Functional Activity (Attached **Annexure-16**):

Impression: _____

_____

Assessment of Environment (Attached **Annexure-17**):

Impression: _____

_____

Other Systems Examination

- Musculoskeletal system:
- Nervous system:
- CVS: DVT/ Postural Dysfunction/Edema:
- GIT:
- Skin: Pressure sore:
- Bladder/Bowel:
    - Retention/Constipation:
    - Autonomous/ Automatic bladder:
- Sexual function:

Diagnostic tests/Special tests (To confirm Diagnosis):

I. Investigation
   - Blood Test
   - Chest X-ray/Radiograph
   - PFT
   - ABG
   - Bronchoscopy
   - Graded exercise test (GXT: Treadmill/Cycle ergometer)
   - Exercise tolerance test
   - 6 min walk test
   - 12 min walk test
   - 10 meter shuttle walk test

Impression: _____

_____

Professional Diagnosis:

Problem list: _____

_____

Management

Short-term Goals

Aims : 1.
        2.
        3.
        4.
        5.

Means : 1.
        2.
        3.
        4.
        5.

Long-term Goals

Aims : 1.
        2.
        3.

Means : 1.
        2.
        3.

Intensive Care Unit Assessment

SUBJECTIVE ASSESSMENT

Demographic Data

Name: _____ Date: _____

Age: _____ Sex: _____

Occupation: _____ Blood Group: _____

Address:

Present: _____ Permanent: _____

_____ _____

_____ _____

_____ _____

Contact No: Res _____ Off: _____

Referring Doctor: _____ Date of Next Visit: _____

Primary Diagnosis: _____

Case History

Chief Complaints: _____

_____

_____

_____

Past Medical History

Date of Onset: _____

Medical History:
- History of Present Condition:
  - Onset of the Condition :
  - Duration of the Condition :
  - Progression of the Symptoms :
- Previous Medical History:
  - Previous Attacks :
  - Previous Treatment :
  - Relevant Medical Condition :

Drug History:
(The drugs which might require alterations in physical therapy treatment)
- Anti-coagulants :
- β-Blockers :
- Bronchodilators :

- Associated Problems:
- Previous Medications:

Medicine	Dosage	Frequency
(i) _____	_____	_____
(ii) _____	_____	_____
(iii) _____	_____	_____

- Previous Surgeries:

Surgery Name	Date	Complication
(i) _____	_____	_____
(ii) _____	_____	_____
(iii) _____	_____	_____

Previous Diagnostic Test Reports:

X- Rays: _____, ECG: _____, P.F.T: _____
ABG: _____, Echo: _____, Blood test: _____
Angiogram: _____, Biochemical test: _____, Others: _____

*General Medical History (Attached **Annexure-1**):*

Personal History

Do you use tobacco products? Alcohol? Recreational drugs? If yes,
- Name and Frequency of Cigarettes/day _____
- Name and Frequency of Alcohol/day _____
- Name and Frequency of Drugs/day _____

Hobbies/Lifestyle: _____
Diet: _____

Family History
- Family background :
- Hereditary complaint :

Occupational History
- Related to present illness :
- Occupational hazards :

Social History:

Examination

1. **Pain Assessment:**
    i. Character of Pain :
    ii. Duration of Pain :
    iii. Location of Pain :
    iv. Behavior of Pain :
    Associated Symptoms (Specify)

2. **Breathlessness:**
    (I – Strenuous activity, II – Ordinary activity, III – < ordinary activity, IV – At rest - NYHA)
    - Dyspnoea Grade:

3. **Cough:**
    - Effectiveness of Cough:
    - Variations in Cough:
    - Productive/Non-Productive:

    Nocturnal Cough – Common in strokes, interstitial lung diseases.
    Productive Cough – Chronic bronchitis, Asthma
    Severe Productive Cough – Early morning, Bronchiectasis

4. **Sputum:**
    i. Colour: Green – Pseudomonas, Black – Smokers, Cold mines, Pink frothy – Pulmonary edema, Bloody – Haemoptysis, Carcinoma, T.B, Bronchiectasis, CHD
    ii. Quantity: Normal – 100 ml/day
    iii. Quality: M1 – Mucoid, M2 – Suspicious about Purulence, M3 – 1/3 Purulent, M4 – 2/3 Purulent, M5 – ¾ Purulent
    iv. Consistency: Mucoid, Purulent, Mucopurulent, Tenacious and Thick
    v. Odor: Foul smelling infection, Bronchiectasis

4. **Wheeze:**
    - Diurnal variations :
    - Positional variations :
    - Aggravating factors :

OBJECTIVE ASSESSMENT

On Observation

A. Level of Consciousness:
   (Alert, Coma, Confused, Paralyzed)

B. Built of the Patient: Ectomorphic/Mesomorphic/Endomorphic
   - Obese with signs of lung obstruction – COPD Type A (Blue Blotters)
   - Thin with signs of lung obstruction – COPD Type B (Pink Buffers)
   - Thin – Chronic infections, T.B, Supportive lesions, Malnutrition, CHD
C. Posture:
   Mention the Level:
   - Thoracotomy – Scoliosis
   - Median Sternotomy – Kyphosis
D. Head and Face evaluation:
   - Facial distress:
   - Cyanotic changes:
E. Neck:
   - Use of accessory muscles – Demand increase
     (Seen in Emphysema and Asthma – Lead to TOS – Because of continuous use of Scalene muscles)
   - Distension of neck veins – In RHF (Distension of Neck veins, Pedal edema, Hepatosplenomegaly)
F. Chest:
   - Unmoving Chest:
     a. Chest wall Deformities – Barrel chest
                                 Pigeon Chest
                                 Funnel Chest
     b. Incision over chest – Extend of Incision
                              Mention drains/Bandages
     c. Any ICD: Upper – Pneumothorax
                 Lower – Effusion
   - Moving Chest:
     a. Symmetry of Movement – Paradoxical or Not
     b. Pattern of Breathing – Rate, Depth, Rhythm
     Euphoria – Normal pattern, Tachypnoea – Increase rate, Bradypnoea – Decrease rate, Hyperpnoea – Increase depth, shallow breathing – in surgery.
     c. Inspiration/Expiration Ratio: 1 . 2 (or) 1: 3
     d. Expansion: Chest wall expansion due to spinal cord injury.
   - Extremity Evaluation:
     1. Clubbing: (In fingers and Toes)
        a. Stages:
        b. Idiopathic reason:
        c. Hypoxemia:
     2. Cyanosis:
        a. Peripheral - (PVD, Nicotine stains)
        b. Central - (Mucosa)
     3. Edema: (Dependent/PVD)
     4. Tremor: (Over use of Bronchodilators)
     5. Skin Changes:
     6. Joint Deformities:

7. External Appliances: (Head to Toe)
    i. Endo Tracheal Tube:
    ii. Ventilator: (rate and mode setting)
    iii. Mask:
    iv. Catheters: (venous and urinary)
    v. Crepe bandage and Stockings:
    vi. Ryle's tube:
- Shape:
    Kyphosis/Kyphoscoliosis/Pectus Excavatum/Pectus Carinatum/Hyperinflation
G. Respiration:
    i. Rate of Respiration :
    ii. Pattern of Respiration:
    Intercostal retraction :
H. Vital Signs:
    Blood pressure   : 120/80 mm Hg
    Respiratory rate : 16-20/min
    Pulse rate   : 72-75
    Temperature   : 98.6°

On Palpation

Trachea:
(A normal trachea may be shifted slightly to the right)
Surgical Emphysema:
1. Tracheal shift (with three fingers):
   (Palpate with middle finger)
   Same side shift: (Atelactasis, Lobectomy, Pneumonectomy) opposite side shift: (Pneumothorax, Pleural effusion, Haemothorax, Haemopneumothorax)
2. Tenderness:
   (From distal site to painful site)
3. Chest Expansion :
   Axillary level   :
   Nipple level   :
   Xiphisternal level :
4. Accessory muscle palpation:
   SCM   :
   Scalene :
5. Tactile fremitus:
   (Ask the patient in sitting position, and ask him to say something.)
   Consolidation: (sound felt distantly)
   Pneumothorax/effusion: (Decreased)
6. Movement of Diaphragm:
   (Thumps under the xiphisternum and ask the patient to inspire and expire and feel the movement of Diaphragm)
7. Pulse:
8. Edema:

9. Capillary filling:
    i. Feel for apex beat. (5th intercostals space, mid-clavicular line, not position and character).
    ii. Feel for heaves (flat of hand over sternum –R-HF, mitral stenosis, pulmonary hypertension).
    iii. Feel for thrills (side of hand horizontal under left clavicle –aortic/ pulmonary stenosis).

On Percussion

- On intercostal suction always compare with other side.
    - Normal – Resonant
    - Air filled areas – Hyper-resonant
    - Consolidated area – Hyporesonant – dull
    - Cardiac dullness 3rd to 5th and 4th to 6th
- Normal Response:
    - Anteriorly   : till 6th rib
    - Laterally   : till 8th rib
    - Posteriorly   : till 10th rib
    (Don't percuss over the scapula)
- Hyper-resonant :
- Normal   :
- Dull   :
- Stony Dull   :

On Auscultation

Lung sounds:
1. Normal sounds:
    a. Tracheal sounds:
        - High pitched sounds
        - Only over trachea
        - Inspiration and Expiration with a pause.
    b. Bronchial sounds:
        - Adjacent to manubrium
        - Not as loud as trachea
        - If this heard over periphery – consolidation
        - Pause between inspiration and expiration
    c. Bronchovesicular:
        - Moderate pitch and intensity
        - Area: Angle of Lewis, between scapula
    d. Vesicular (Breath sounds)
        - Very soft and muffled breeze through leaves
        - Heard due to Turbulence
        - Pause decreases
        - Heard in all Peripheral areas
        - Air is not entering from central to periphery (Pneumothorax, Effusion)
        - Hyperinflated lung (Asthma)
        - Any Obstruction – complete absence

2. Voice Sounds: (Same as tactile fremitus)
   - Bronchophony – 99,123 etc
   - Egophony – E to A (Say E, E – hear as 'A')
   - Whispering pectoriloquy:
     - Whispering only
     - Normally nothing is heard
     - In consolidation – Distinct sound heard
3. Added sounds:
   a. Wheeze/Bronchi:
      - Air coming through the obstructed pathway
      - Musical and Rhythmic
      - Bronchospasm (Asthma)
      - Common in expiration
      - Heard both during inspiration and expiration
      - Chronic bronchitis
   b. Crepitations/Rales:
      - Due to secretions
      - Opening of closed Airways
      - Heard clearly during deep inspiration

- Lung sounds :
- Added sounds:
- Heart sounds :
   i. First screen; whilst palpating CA, listen in all 4 regions with both bell and diaphragm, noting no. of heart sounds (s3 norm. in most cases, s4 always abnormal.) and any additional sounds.
   ii. 4 Regions – Aortic (2nd ICS, RSE), Pulmonary (2nd ICS, LSE), Tricuspid (4th ICS, LSE, pt leaning forward, breath held in exp.),
   Mitral (4th ICS, MCL). also Mitral regurgitation. (pt on L side, listen medial to axillary line), apex (5th ICS, MCL).
   iii. If suspected murmur
   iv. Describe as:
      1. Systolic/Diastolic.
      2. Ejection/Pansystolic.
      3. High/Low.
      4. Grade 1-4.
      5. Influence of respiration (L sided murmurs are increased on expiration and R sided decreased).
      6. Radiation (carotids in aortic stenosis, axilla in mitral regurg.).
      7. Influence of rolling on L side (mitral stenosis at the apex).
      8. On sitting forward in expiration (aortic regurg. and stenosis).

Inspection

General appearance—
i. Scars (sternotomy, valvotomy) or dilated veins.
ii. Visible pulsation/heaves.
iii. Pectus excavatum (Marfan's syndrome).

i. **Postural Alignment:**
   Impression: _____

ii. **Contour and Alignment of Bone and Joints:**
    Impression: _____

iii. **Size and Contour of Soft Tissue Structure:**
     Impression: _____

iv. **Size and Contour of Nails:**
    _____

Colour and Texture of Skin and Tongue

Cyanosis: _____	Pallor: _____
Erythema (localized, generalized): _____	Yellow skin: _____
Highly pigmented hairy areas: _____	Open wounds: _____
Scars: New scar: _____	Old scar: _____

Thickening, thinning, and hair loss: _____

Palpation

i. **Bony Prominences (Pain, Abnormal Alignment):**
   Antr Surface: _____
   Postr Surface: _____
   Lat Surface: (Rt) _____ (Lt) _____

ii. **Soft Tissue Structures:**

Pain: _____	Tenderness Grade: _____
Swelling: _____	Spasm: _____
Nodules: _____	Trigger points: _____
Fascia tightness: _____	Mobility of Soft tissue: _____

Density and Extensibility of soft tissues: _____

Tenderness grade:
1: Patient feels pain
2: Patient winces
3: Patient winces and withdraws
4: Patient won't allow to touch

Impression: _____

iii. **Skin:**

Warmth: _____	Density: _____
Extensibility of skin: _____	Peripheral pulses: _____
Edema (pitting or non-pitting edema): _____	Grade: _____

Anthropometric Measurements

1. Limb length: (i) True length: (Rt) _____ (Lt) _____
   (ii) Apparent length: (Rt) _____ (Lt) _____
2. Circumference Measurement:
   - Upper arm :
   - Forearm :
   - Mid-thigh :
   - Calf :
   - Chest :

Examination of the Hands

a. Peripheral cyanosis (colour, temperature and sweat).
b. Clubbing (cyanotic congenital heart disease, infective endocarditis, atrial myxoma).
c. Splinter haemorrhages (5+ on one hand is significant. Check occupation. May suggest infective endocarditis).
d. Capillary refill time (press for 5 secs).
e. Tendon xanthomata (fatty deposits in tendons - hyperlipidaemia).
f. Anaemia (check palmar creases for colour).
g. Osler's nodes (painful swellings on tips of fingers, suggestive of infective endocarditis).
h. Janeaway lesions (small red pimples on pulps of hands. Differentiated from Osler's by; being painless and blanching on compression).
i. Tar stains (white fatty deposits on palms).
j. Rheumatoid signs (ulnar deviation, swan neck and suggestive of multisystem disease).

Examination of the Radial Pulse

a. Rate and rhythm (norm. rate is 60-100 bpm. Irregularly irregular suggests AF. Regularly irregular suggests second degree heart block).
b. Radio-radial delay (delay of L radial compared to R – coarctation of the aorta proximal to the L subclavian artery).
c. Radio-femoral delay (coarctation of the aorta).
d. Collapsing pulse (water-hammer – aortic regurgitation, patent ductus arteriosus).

Examination of the Brachial Artery

a. blood pressure;
   i. Both sitting and standing (>15/20 mm Hg difference – orthostatic/postural hypotension).
   ii. In right and left arm (>10 mm Hg difference is a sign of aortic dissection or coarctation of the aorta. Make a note to always use the arm that gives the higher reading).

Examination of the Carotid Artery

a. Assess character and volume.
b. Low volume, plateau pulse and slow rising (aortic stenosis).
c. Rapid upstroke and down stroke (aortic regurgitation).
d. Auscultate for bruits, moving the diaphragm up the artery (atherosclerosis, aortic stenosis).

Examination of JVP (Jugular Venous Pressure)

a. Measure vertical height (cm) from sternal angle to top of jugular venous pulsation. Norm. is 7 mm Hg,–no more than 4 cm above s.a.
b. If difficulty finding JVP, apply abdominal pressure for 5-10 secs (hepatojugular reflux) to amplify its presence.
c. Can be distinguished from the carotid pulse commonly by its double peaked wave form (right atrial contraction and atrial filling during ventricular systole) and also by palpation.
d. Elevated JVP in R-sided HF, PE, pericardial effusion/constriction and sup. vena caval obstruction. Altered wave pulsation in – AF, tricuspid stenosis/regurgitation, complete heart block. (NB. Can also be elevated in pregnancy, fluid overload hypertension, Kussmaul's sign – cardiac tamponade).

Examine the Face

a. General:
i. Colour, temperature, sweat.
ii. Malar flush (cheeks – mitral stenosis).

b. Eyes:
i. Corneal arcus (cholesterol crystals in periphery of cornea. In young associated with hypercholesterolaemia, association weakens with age –arcus senilis).
ii. Xanthelasma (hyperlipidaemia).
iii. Anaemia (bottom eyelid).
iv. Jaundice (sclera).

c. Tongue:
i. Central cyanosis (under tongue).
ii. Dentition (infective endocarditis).

Examine the Chest (NB. Dextrocardia possible!):

1. **Range of Motion** (Attached **Annexure-3**):
   (Find the Amount, Quality, Pattern, Pain and Crepitus) AROM, PROM
   Impression: _____

2. **Muscle Strength Assessment** (Attached **Annexure-6**):
   Impression: _____

3. **Muscle Length Assessment** (Attached **Annexure-7**):
   Impression: _____

4. **Assessment of Sensation** (Attached **Annexure-8**):
   Superficial: _____

   Deep: _____

5. **Assessment of Reflex** (Attached **Annexure-9**):
   Superficial: _____
   _____

   Deep: _____
   _____

6. **Assessment of Posture** (Attached **Annexure-14**):
   Impression: _____
   _____
   _____

7. **External Devices Used:**
   Impression: _____
   _____
   _____

8. **Other Systems Examination:**
   - Musculoskeletal system:
   - Nervous system:
   - Automatic:
   - CVS: DVT/Postural Dysfunction/Edema:
   - Respiratory system:
     - Type/Pattern of Breathing:
     - Chest expansion: Symmetrical or Asymmetrical:
     - Chest deformities:
   - GIT:
   - Skin: Pressure sore:
   - Bladder/Bowel:
     - Retention:
     - Constipation:
     - Autonomous/Automatic bladder:
   - Sexual function:

Diagnostic tests/Special tests (To confirm Diagnosis):
I. Investigation
   - Blood Test
   - Chest X-ray/Radiograph
   - PFT
   - ABG
- Bronchoscopy

Impression: _____
_____

Professional Diagnosis:
Problem list: _____
_____
_____

Management

Short-term Goals

Aims : 1.
        2.
        3.

Means : 1.
         2.
         3.

Long-term Goals

Aims : 1.
        2.
        3.

Means : 1.
         2.
         3.

13 CHAPTER

Geriatric Assessment

SUBJECTIVE ASSESSMENT

Demographic Data

Name: _____ Date: _____

Age: _____ Sex: _____

Occupation: _____

Address:

Present: _____ Permanent: _____
_____ _____
_____ _____
_____ _____

Contact No.: Res _____ Off: _____

Referring Doctor: _____ Date of Next Visit: _____

Primary Diagnosis: _____

Case History

Chief Complaints: _____
_____
_____
_____

Past Medical History

Date of Onset: _____
_____
_____
_____

Medical History Questionnaire

1. What previous care has been sought for the problem?
2. Who else has treated the problem?
3. What tests and treatment did they perform?
4. What have you done to relieve the problem?
5. Has this problem occurred before? If yes, how was it treated or resolved?
   i. Previous Medications:

Medicine	Dosage	Frequency
(i) _____	_____	_____
(ii) _____	_____	_____
(iii) _____	_____	_____

   ii. Previous Surgeries:

Surgery Name	Date	Complication
(i) _____	_____	_____
(ii) _____	_____	_____
(iii) _____	_____	_____

   iii. Previous Diagnostic Test Reports:

   X- rays: _____, C.T Scan: _____, M.R.I: _____

   Bone scan: _____, EMG: _____, Blood test: _____

   Myelogram: _____, Biochemical test: _____, Others: _____

Drug Allergy

Able to take medication by herself or himself:

General Medical History (Attached **Annexure-1**):

Personal History

Do you use tobacco products? Alcohol? Recreational drugs? If yes,
- Name and Frequency of Cigarettes/day _____
- Name and Frequency of Alcohol/day _____
- Name and Frequency of Drugs/day _____
    i. What percentage of your normal work activities are you able to perform?
       0% 10% 20% 30% 40% 50% 60% 70% 80% 90% 100%
    ii. What percentage of your normal home activities are you able to perform?
       0% 10% 20% 30% 40% 50% 60% 70% 80% 90% 100%
    iii. What percentage of your normal recreational activities are you able to perform?
       0% 10% 20% 30% 40% 50% 60% 70% 80% 90% 100%

Family History
- Family Background:
- Hereditary Complaint:

Occupational History
- Related to present illness:
- Occupational hazards for illness:

Social History
i. Do you live alone and what type of work do you do in and outside of the home?
ii. How has this problem affected your ability to perform your job?
iii. Do you have to climb stairs to get into your house? Reach the bedroom?
iv. Level of Involvement with the community.

Economic History
1. Onset of Pain:
   a. Sudden: Yes/No, If yes how? _____
   b. Gradual: Yes/No, If yes how? _____
   c. Congenital onset: Yes/No, If yes how? _____
2. Location of Pain (Through body chart)

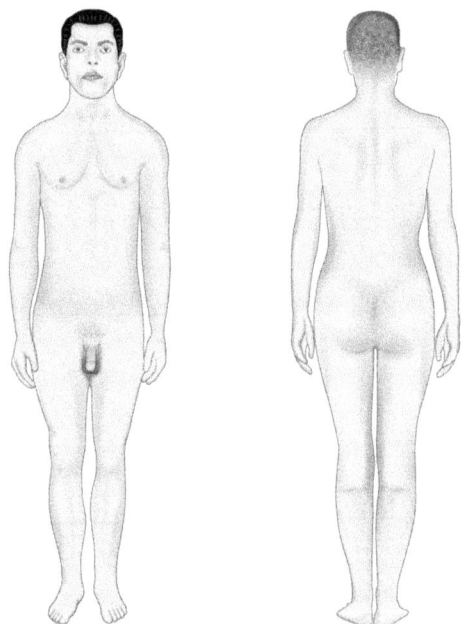

   - Has the pain change in location: Yes/No, if yes, where _____
   - Spread to other areas: Yes/No, if yes, where _____
   - Become more focused: Yes/No, if yes, where _____
3. Intensity of Pain: (Ask the patient to rate his or her pain in this scale.)
   Visual Analog scale:

   No pain   Pain as bad as it could possibly be
4. Type of pain (Attached **Annexure-2**):

5. Behavior of symptoms:
   What makes your symptoms increase?
   i. Rest: yes/no, if yes, which position _____
   ii. Activity: yes/no, if yes, which position _____
   iii. Body position: yes/no, if yes, which position _____
   What makes your symptoms decrease?
   i. Rest: yes/no, if yes, which position _____
   ii. Activity: yes/no, if yes, which position _____
   iii. Body position: yes/no, if yes, which position _____
   Behavior of symptom during the last 48 hours:
   Better, worse, staying the same: _____

Recognizing Pain Patterns:

Indicate a plus (+) for aggravating factors or a minus (−) for relieving factors

Liquor	Sleep/rest
Stimulants (e.g. caffeine)	Lying down
Eating	Distraction (e.g.) television
Heat	Urination/Defecation
Cold	Tension/Stress
Weather changes	Loud noise
Massage	Going to work
Pressure	Intercourse
No movement	Mild Exercise
Movement	Fatigue
Sitting	Standing

OBJECTIVE ASSESSMENT

Mental Status

1. Level of consciousness :
2. Orientation to
   i. Person :
   ii. Place :
   iii. Time :
3. General arousal state :
4. Cognitive state :
5. Communication ability :
6. Vital signs:
   – Blood pressure (standing/Lying) : 120/80 mm Hg
   – Orthostatic blood pressure :
   – Respiratory rate : 16-20/min
   – Pulse rate : 72-75
   – Temperature : 98.6°F

Observation

- Apparent age: _____
- State of health: _____
- Nutritional status: _____
- General posture: _____
- Ability to perform status: _____
- Changing the position: _____
- Transfer from sitting to standing: _____
- Ambulate to the examining room: _____
- Built of the patient: Ectomorphic/Mesomorphic/Endomorphic

Ideal Body Weight (IBW)

- For females: 45.5 kg + (2.3 kg) (each inch of height >5 feet)
- For males: 50 kg + (2.3 kg) (each inch of height >5 feet)

Lean Body Mass

- LBW: 0.4 (actual body weight - IBW)
- BMI : Weight (kg)/height^2(m)

Inspection

i. **Postural Alignment:**

   a. Anterior view:

Both eyes: _____	Acromian process: _____
Iliac crests: _____	ASIS: _____
Greater trochanter: _____	Patellae: _____
Ankle malleoli: _____	Waist angle: _____

   b. Posterior view:

Earlobes: _____	Spine of the scapula: _____
Shoulder: _____	Inferior angle of scapula: _____
Iliac crests: _____	PSIS: _____
Greater trochanter: _____	Buttocks: _____
Knee creases: _____	Ankle malleoli: _____
Spine: _____	

ii. **Lateral view** (see through the line of gravity – Impression): _____
   _____

iii. **Contour and Alignment of Bone and Joints:**
   Impression: _____
   _____

iv. **Size and Contour of Soft Tissue Structure:**
   Soft tissue edema: _____ Joint effusion: _____
   Muscle hypertrophy: _____ Muscle atrophy: _____
   Muscle rupture: _____ Cysts, Rheumatoid nodules: _____
   Ganglion: _____ Gouty tophi: _____
   Impression: _____

v. **Size and Contour of Nails:**
   _____
   _____
   Clubbing (Grade): _____

vi. **Colour and Texture of Skin and Tongue:**
   Cyanosis: _____ Pallor: _____
   Erythema (localized, generalized): _____ Yellow skin: _____
   Highly pigmented hairy areas: _____ Open wounds: _____
   Scars: New scar: _____ Old scar: _____
   Thickening, thinning, and hair loss: _____

Palpation

i. Bony Prominences (Pain, Abnormal Alignment):
   Antr Surface: _____
   Postr Surface: _____
   Lat Surface: (Rt) _____ (Lt) _____

ii. Soft Tissue Structures:
   Pain: _____ Tenderness Grade: _____
   Swelling: _____ Spasm: _____
   Nodules: _____ Trigger points: _____
   Fascia tightness: _____ Mobility of soft tissue: _____
   Density and Extensibility of soft tissues: _____
   Impression: _____

iii. Skin:
   Warmth: _____ Density: _____
   Extensibility of skin: _____ Peripheral pulses: _____
   Edema (pitting or non-pitting edema): ___ Grade: _____

Anthropometric Measurements

1. Limb length: (i) True length: (Rt) _____ (Lt) _____
                (ii) Apparent length: (Rt) _____ (Lt) _____

2. Circumference Measurement:
   Upper arm: Rt _____ Lt _____
   Forearm   : Rt _____ Lt _____
   Mid-thigh : Rt _____ Lt _____
   Calf   : Rt _____ Lt _____
   Chest   : _____

Examination

1. **Assessment of Mental Status** mini-cog assessment instrument:
   Impression: _____

2. **Assessment of Emotional Status** Geriatric Depression Scale:
   Impression: _____

3. **Assessment of Range of Motion** (Attached **Annexure-3**):
   (Find the Amount, Quality, Pattern, Pain and Crepitus) AROM, PROM
   Impression: _____

4. **Assessment of Muscle Strength Assessment** (Attached **Annexure-6**):
   Impression: _____

5. **Assessment of Muscle Length Assessment** (Attached **Annexure-7**):
   Impression: _____

6. **Assessment of Sensation** (Attached **Annexure-8**):
   Superficial: _____

   Deep: _____

7. **Assessment of Posture** (Attached **Annexure-14**):
   Impression: _____

8. **Assessment of Gait** (Attached **Annexure-15**):
   Performance-oriented mobility assessment (POMA)

Distance walked	Step length difference
Elapsed time	Cadence
Walking velocity	Width of walking base
Left stride length	Left foot angle
Right stride length	Right foot angle
Left step length	Right stride length to Right L.L length
Right step length	Left stride length to Left L.L length

Impression: _____

9. **Assessment of Function** (Attached **Annexure-16**):
   Philadelphia Geriatric Center Multilevel Assessment Instrument

   Impression: _____

10. **Assessment of Environment** (Attached **Annexure-17**):

    Impression: _____

11. **Assessment of Nutritional Status** (Attached **Annexure-24**):

    Impression: _____

12. **External Devices Used:**

    Impression: _____

13. **Other Systems Examination:**
    - Nervous system:
    - CVS: DVT/Postural Dysfunction/Edema:
      - Apical impulse, rate and rhythm:
      - Heart sounds, murmurs, rubs and gallops:
    - Respiratory system: Type/Pattern of Breathing:
      - Chest expansion/Chest deformities:
      - Percussion/Auscultation:
    - Skin: Pressure sore:
    - Vision: Snellen chart or Jaeger chart
    - Hearing:
    - Oral cavity: No. of teeth, loose teeth, caries
    - Bladder/Bowel: Retention/Constipation/Autonomous/Automatic bladder:
    - Sexual function:
    - Physical diagnosis:
    - Functional diagnosis:

Professional Diagnosis:
Problem list: _____

Management

Short-term Goals

Aims : 1.
        2.
        3.
Means : 1.
         2.
         3.

Long-term Goals

Aims : 1.
        2.
        3.
Means : 1.
         2.
         3.

ANNEXURES

Annexure 1

General Medical History—Questionnaire

Do you have, or have you had any of the following: Please check all that apply

- High Blood Pressure
- Heart Problems
- Heart Palpitations, Murmur
- Thyroid Problems
- Shortness of Breath
- Coughing
- Dialysis
- Blood Transfusion
- Asthma
- Allergies
- Changes in Hair/Nail
- Any Fracture
- Any Supportive Devices
- Hip/Ankle Problem
- Loss of Appetite
- Incontinence
- Abnormal/Painful Menstruation
- Pelvic Inflammation Disease

- Hot/Cold Intolerance
- Diabetes
- Low Blood Sugar
- Seizures
- Tumors/Cancer
- Bleeding/Bruising
- Balance Problems
- Lung Problems
- Rashes
- Scars
- Joint/Muscle Pain
- Recent Wt Gain or Loss
- Nausea or Vomiting
- Bowel or Bladder Changes
- Blood in Urine
- Sexual Dysfunction
- Vocal Changes
- Difficulty in Eating

- Dentures
- Major Dental Work
- Chest Pain
- Head Trauma, Paralysis
- Headache
- Dizziness
- Difficulty in Sleeping
- Arthritis
- Varicose Vein
- Muscle Cramp
- Ulcers
- Wear Eye Glasses/Lens
- Changes in Vision
- Blurred/Double Vision
- Difficulty in Swallowing
- Ear Pain
- Psychiatric Problems
- Psychological Problems

2 Annexure

Type of Pain History—Questionnaire

Do you have, or have you had any of the following type of pain.

Vascular	Neurogenic	Emotional
Throbbing	Stabbing	Tiring
Pounding	Crushing	Miserable
Pulsing	Pinching	Vicious
Beating	Burning	Agonizing
Musculoskeletal	Hot	Nauseating
Aching	Searing	Frightful
Sore	Itching	Piercing
Heavy	Pulling	Dreadful
Hurting	Jumping	Punishing
Dull	Shooting	Torturing
	Pricking	Killing
	Gnawing	Unbearable
		Annoying
		Stinging

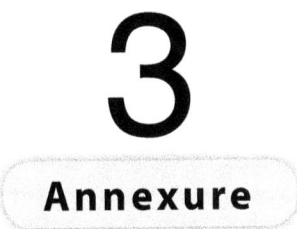

Assessment of Range of Motion

Right		Range of Motion	Left	
AROM	PROM		AROM	PROM
		TM Joint		
		Depression		
		Anterior Protrusion		
		Lateral Deviation		
		Cervical Spine		
		Flexion (40)		
		Extension (50)		
		Lateral Flexion (45)		
		Rotation (90)		
		Thoracolumbar Spine		
		Flexion (40)		
		Extension (30)		
		Lateral Flexion (35)		
		Rotation (45)		
		Lumbar Spine		
		Flexion (35)		
		Extension (55)		
		Lateral Flexion (45)		
		Rotation (45)		
		Hip		
		Flexion (120)		
		Extension (20)		
		Abduction (45)		
		Adduction (10)		
		Medial Rotation (45)		
		Lateral Rotation (45)		
		Knee		
		Flexion (145)		
		Extension (0)		

Contd...

Contd...

Right		Range of Motion	Left	
AROM	PROM		AROM	PROM
		Ankle		
		Plantar Flexion (45)		
		Dorsi Flexion (20)		
		Inversion (25)		
		Eversion (15)		
		Foot		
		1st MTP Flexion (45)		
		1st MTP Extension (50)		
		1st MTP Abduction		
		1st IP Flexion (90)		
		MTP Flexion (90)		
		MTP Extension (50)		
		MTP Abduction		
		PIP Flexion (65)		
		DIP Flexion (30)		
		DIP Extension (0)		
		Shoulder		
		Flexion (180)		
		Extension (60)		
		Abduction (180)		
		Medial Rotation (70)		
		Lateral Rotation (90)		
		Elbow & Forearm		
		Flexion (145)		
		Extension (0)		
		Supination (90)		
		Pronation (90)		
		Wrist		
		Flexion (80)		
		Extension (70)		
		Ulnar Deviation (45)		
		Radial Deviation (20)		
		Thumb		
		CMC Flexion (15)		
		CMC Extension (20)		
		CMC Abduction (60)		
		CMC Opposition		
		MCP Flexion (50)		
		IP Flexion (80)		
		IP Extension (20)		

Contd...

Contd...

Right		Range of Motion	Left	
AROM	PROM		AROM	PROM
		Index Finger		
		MCP Flexion (90)		
		MCP Extension (45)		
		MCP Abduction (20)		
		PIP Flexion (100)		
		DIP Flexion (90)		
		Middle Finger		
		MCP Flexion (90)		
		MCP Extension (45)		
		MCP Abduction (20)		
		PIP Flexion (100)		
		DIP Flexion (90)		
		Ring Finger		
		MCP Flexion (90)		
		MCP Extension (45)		
		PIP Flexion (100)		
		DIP Flexion (90)		
		Little Finger		
		MCP Flexion (90)		
		MCP Extension (45)		
		PIP Flexion (100)		
		DIP Flexion (90)		

4
Annexure

Assessment of End Feel

F – Firm, S – Soft, H – Hard

Right	End Feel	Left
	TM Joint	
	Depression (F)	
	Anterior Protrusion (F)	
	Lateral Deviation (F)	
	Cervical Spine	
	Flexion (F)	
	Extension (F)	
	Lateral Flexion (F)	
	Rotation (F)	
	Thoracolumbar Spine	
	Flexion (F)	
	Extension (F)	
	Lateral Flexion (F)	
	Rotation (F)	
	Lumbar Spine	
	Flexion (F)	
	Extension (F)	
	Lateral Flexion (F)	
	Rotation (F)	
	Hip	
	Flexion (S)	
	Extension (F)	
	Abduction (F)	
	Adduction (F)	
	Medial Rotation (F)	
	Lateral Rotation (F)	
	Knee	
	Flexion (S)	
	Extension (F)	

Contd...

Contd...

Right	End Feel	Left
	Ankle	
	Plantar Flexion (F)	
	Dorsi Flexion (F)	
	Inversion (F)	
	Eversion (H)	
	Foot	
	1st MTP Flexion (F)	
	1st MTP Extension (F)	
	1st MTP Abduction (F)	
	1st IP Flexion (S)	
	MTP Flexion (F)	
	MTP Extension (F)	
	MTP Abduction (F)	
	PIP Flexion (S)	
	DIP Flexion (F)	
	DIP Extension (F)	
	Shoulder	
	Flexion (F)	
	Extension (F)	
	Abduction (F)	
	Medial Rotation (F)	
	Lateral Rotation (F)	
	Elbow & Forearm	
	Flexion (S)	
	Extension (H)	
	Supination (F)	
	Pronation (H)	
	Wrist	
	Flexion (F)	
	Extension (F)	
	Ulnar Deviation (F)	
	Radial Deviation (H)	
	Thumb	
	CMC Flexion (S)	
	CMC Extension (F)	
	CMC Abduction (F)	
	CMC Opposition (S)	
	MCP Flexion (H)	
	IP Flexion (F)	
	IP Extension (F)	
	Index Finger	
	MCP Flexion (H)	
	MCP Extension (F)	
	MCP Abduction (F)	
	PIP Flexion (H)	
	DIP Flexion (F)	

Contd...

Contd...

Right	End Feel	Left
	Middle Finger	
	MCP Flexion (H)	
	MCP Extension (F)	
	MCP Abduction (F)	
	PIP Flexion (H)	
	DIP Flexion (F)	
	Ring Finger	
	MCP Flexion (H)	
	MCP Extension (F)	
	PIP Flexion (H)	
	DIP Flexion (F)	
	Little Finger	
	MCP Flexion (H)	
	MCP Extension (F)	
	PIP Flexion (H)	
	DIP Flexion (F)	

5
Annexure

Assessment of Capsular Pattern of Restriction

Joints	Proportional Limitations	Comments
TM Joint	Limitation of mouth opening	
Atlanto-occipital	Forward bending > Backward bending	
Atlantoaxial	Restriction with rotation	
Lower cervical spine	Rotation > backward bending	
Sternoclavicular	Pain at extreme range of motion	
Acromioclavicular	Pain at extreme range of motion	
Glenohumeral	Ext. Rot > Abd > Int. Rot	
Humeroulnar	Flexion > Extension	
Humeroradial	Flexion > Extension	
Prox & Dist radioulnar	Pronation = Supinaton	
Wrist	Flexion = Extension	
Midcarpal	Limitation in all directions	
Carpometacarpal II - V	Limitation in all directions	
All PIP and DIP	Flexion > Extension	
Thoracic spine	Side bending > Extension > Flexion	
Cervical spine	Side bending > Extension > Flexion	
Sacroiliac	Pain when joints are stressed	
Hip	Flexion > Int. Rot > Abduction	
Knee	Flexion > Extension	
Tibiofibular	Pain when joints are stressed	
Talocrural	Plantar flexion > Dorsiflexion	
Talocalcaneal	Inversion > Eversion	
Midtarsal	Supination > Pronation	
I st MTP	Extension > Flexion	
MTP (II – V)	Flexion restrictions	
Interphalangeal	Extension restrictions	

6 Annexure

Assessment of Muscle Strength

Right	Muscle Strength	Left
	Neck	
	Capital Extensors	
	Cervical Extensors	
	Combined Extensors	
	Capital Flexors	
	Cervical Flexors	
	Combined Flexors	
	Cervical Rotators	
	Trunk	
	Extensors – Lumbar	
	Extensors – Thoracic	
	Flexors	
	Rotators	
	Pelvic Elevators	
	Hip	
	Hip Flexors	
	Hip Extensors	
	Hip Abductors	
	Hip Adductors	
	Hip External Rotators	
	Hip Internal Rotators	
	Knee	
	Knee Flexors	
	Knee Extensors	
	Ankle & Foot	
	Ankle Plantar Flexors	
	Ankle Dorsi Flexors	
	Foot Invertors	
	Foot Evertors	
	1st Toe MCP Flexors	
	1st Toe MCP Extensors	
	1st Toe IP Flexors	
	1st Toe IP Extensors	
	Toe MCP Flexors	

Contd...

Contd...

Right	Muscle Strength	Left
	Toe MCP Extensors	
	Toe IP Flexors	
	Toe IP Extensors	
	Upper Extremity	
	Shoulder	
	Scapular Abductors	
	Scapular Adductors	
	Scapular Elevators	
	Shoulder Flexors	
	Shoulder Extensors	
	Shoulder Scaptors	
	Shoulder Abductors	
	Horizontal Abductors	
	Horizontal Adductors	
	External Rotators	
	Internal Rotators	
	Elbow & Forearm	
	Elbow Flexors	
	Elbow Extensors	
	Forearm Supinators	
	Forearm Pronators	
	Wrist	
	Wrist Flexors	
	Wrist Extensors	
	Hand & Fingers	
	Finger MCP Flexors	
	Finger MCP Extensors	
	Finger PIP Flexors	
	Finger DIP Flexors	
	Finger Abductors	
	Finger Adductors	
	Thumb MCP Flexors	
	Thumb MCP Extensors	
	Thumb IP Flexors	
	Thumb IP Extensors	
	Thumb Abductors	
	Thumb Adductors	
	Thumb Oppositors	

7
Annexure

Assessment of Muscle Length

Right	Muscle Length	Left
	Upper Extremity	
	Pectoralis Major	
	Pectoralis Minor	
	Biceps Brachi	
	Triceps Brachi	
	Flexor Digitorum Superficialis	
	Flexor Digitorum Profundus	
	Palmaris Longus	
	Flexor Carpi Radialis	
	Flexor Carpi Ulnaris	
	Extensor Digitorum	
	Extensor Carpi Radialis Longus/Brevis	
	Extensor Carpi Ulnaris	
	Lumbricals	
	Palmar Fascia	
	Lower Extremity	
	Psoas Major	
	Rectus Femoris	
	Sartorius	
	Biceps Femoris	
	Tensor Fascia Lata	
	Gastrocnemius	
	Soleus	
	Plantar Fascia	
	Spine	
	Sternocleidomastoid	
	Splenius Capitis	
	Levator Scapulae	
	Rhomboidus Major	
	Rhomboidus Minor	
	Lumbar Fascia	

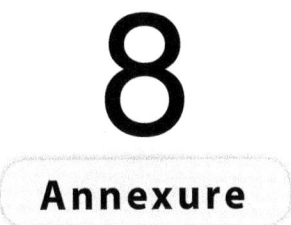

Assessment of Sensation

Key to Grading:
1. **Intact:** Normal accurate response
2. **Decreased:** Delayed response
3. **Exaggerated:** Increased sensitivity or awareness of stimulus after removal
4. **Inaccurate:** Inappropriate perception of stimulus
5. **Absent:** No response
6. **Inconsistent or Ambiguous:** Response inadequate to determine function accurately

Sensation (U.E)	Right	Left	Comments
Pain			
Temperature			
Touch			
Vibration			
2– point Discrimination			
Kinesthesia			
Proprioception			
Stereognosis			

Sensation (L.E)	Right	Left	Comments
Pain			
Temperature			
Touch			
Vibration			
2 – point Discrimination			
Kinesthesia			
Proprioception			

Sensation (Trunk)	Right	Left	Comments
Pain			
Temperature			
Touch			
Vibration			
2 – point Discrimination			

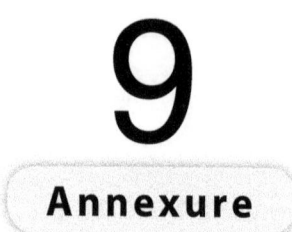

Assessment of Reflex

Superficial Reflex:

Reflex	Normal Response	Patient's Response
Upper abdominal	Umbilicus moves up and toward area being stroked	
Lower abdominal	Umbilicus moves down and toward area being stroked	
Cremastric	Scrotum elevates	
Plantar	Flexion of toes	
Gluteal	Skin tenses in gluteal area	
Anal	Contraction of anal sphincter muscles	

Deep Tendon Reflex:

Reflex	Normal Response	Patient's Response
Jaw	Mouth closes	
Biceps	Biceps contraction	
Brachioradialis	Flexion of elbow and/or pronation of forearm	
Triceps	Elbow extension and muscle contraction	
Patella	Leg extension	
Medial Hamstrings	Knee flexion and muscle contraction	
Lateral Hamstrings	Knee flexion and muscle contraction	
Tibialis Posterior	Plantar flexion of foot	
Achilles	Plantar flexion of foot	

10

Annexure

Assessment of Non-equilibrium

NON-EQUILIBRIUM TESTS

Key to Grading:
5 – **Normal Performance**
4 – **Minimal Impairment:** Able to accomplish: slightly less than normal speed; requires supervision/ minimal contact guarding.
3 – **Moderate Impairment:** Able to accomplish activity: movements are slow, awkward, and unsteady; requires moderate guarding.
2 – **Severe Impairment:** Able only to initiate activity without completion; requires maximal contact guarding.
1 – **Activity Impossible**

Grade (Rt)	Co-ordination Test	Grade (Lt)	Comments
	Finger-to-nose		
	Finger-to-therapist's finger		
	Finger-to-finger		
	Alternate nose-to-finger		
	Finger opposition		
	Mass grasp		
	Pronation/Supination		
	Rebound phenomenon		
	Tapping (hand)		
	Tapping (foot)		
	Pointing and past-pointing		
	Alternate heel-to-knee, heel-to-toe		
	Toe-to-examiner's finger		
	Heel-on-shin		
	Drawing a circle (hand)		
	Drawing a circle (foot)		
	Fixation/position holding (UE)		
	Fixation/position holding (LE)		

Notations should be made under comments section if,
- Lack of visual input renders activity impossible or alters quality of performance.
- Verbal cuing is required to accomplish activity.
- Alterations in speed affect quality of performance
- Excessive amount of time required to complete activity
- Changes in arm position alters sitting balance
- Extraneous movements, unsteadiness, or oscillations noted in head, neck, or trunk.

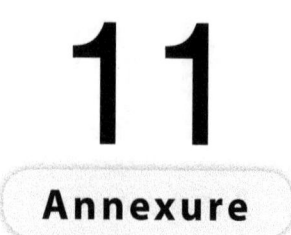

Assessment of Equilibrium

EQUILIBRIUM COORDINATION TESTS

Key to Grading:
5 – **Normal Performance**
4 – **Minimal Impairment:** Able to accomplish: slightly less than normal speed; requires supervision/ minimal contact guarding.
3 – **Moderate Impairment:** Able to accomplish activity: movements are slow, awkward, and unsteady; requires moderate guarding.
2 – **Severe Impairment:** Able only to initiate activity without completion; requires maximal contact guarding.
1 – **Activity Impossible**

Coordination Test	Grade	Comments
Standing in a normal comfortable posture		
Standing feet together		
Standing on one foot		
Standing with one foot in front of other-tandem position		
Standing, forward trunk flexion and return to normal		
Standing, laterally flex trunk to each side		
Standing eyes open to eyes closed – Romberg test		
Standing in tandem position. Eyes open to eyes closed		
Walk at normal speed		
Walk as fast as possible		
Walk as slow as possible		
Walk: stop and start abruptly		
Walk and pivot (turn 90, 180, or 360 degree)		
Tandem walking		
Walking along a straight line		
Walking, placing feet on floor markers		
Walk – sideways, Backwards		
Walk – cross- stepping		
Walk – in a circle, alternate directions		
Walk – on heels		
Walk – on toes		
March in place		
Walk with horizontal and vertical head turns		
Step over or around obstacles		
Stair climbing: with handrail		
Stair climbing: without handrail		
Stair climbing: one step at a time		
Stair climbing: step over step		

12
Annexure

Assessment of Dermatome

Nerve Root	Dermatome	Patient Response
C1	Vertex of Skull	
C2	Temple, forehead, Occiput	
C3	Entire neck, Posterior cheek, temporal area, prolongation Forward under mandible.	
C4	Shoulder area, clavicular area Upper scapular area	
C5	Deltoid area, Anterior aspect Of entire arm to base of thumb.	
C6	Anterior arm, Radial side of hand To thumb and index finger.	
C7	Lateral arm and forearm to Index Long and ring fingers.	
C8	Medial arm and forearm to long, Ring and little fingers.	
T1	Medial side of forearm to base of little finger	
T2	Medial side of upper arm to Medial elbow, pectoral and mid-scapular areas	
T3 – T12	T3-T6, Upper thorax, T5-T7, costal margin, T8-T12 abdomen and Lumbar region	
L1	Back over trochanter and groin	
L2	Back, front of thigh to knee	
L3	Back, upper buttock, anterior thigh and knee, medial lower leg	
L4	Medial buttock, lateral thigh, medial leg, dorsum of foot, big toe	
L5	Buttock, posterior and lateral thigh Lateral aspect of leg, dorsum of foot, medial half of sole, first, Second and third toes.	
S1	Buttock, thigh, and leg posterior	
S2	Same as S1	
S3	Groin, medial thigh to knee	
S4	Peroneun, genitals, lower sacrum	

13 Annexure

Assessment of Myotome

Nerve Root	Myotome	Patient Response
C1	Upper cervical flexion	
	Rectus capitis anterior, lateralis, posterior	
C2	Upper cervical extension	
	Longus colli, Rectus capitis	
C3	Cervical lateral flexion	
	Trapezius, Splenius capitis	
C4	Shoulder shrugging	
	Trapezius, Levator Scapulae	
C5	Shoulder abduction, External rotation	
	Supraspinatus, Deltoid, Infraspinatus	
	Biceps	
C6	Elbow flexion, Wrist extension	
	Biceps, Supinator, Wrist extensors	
C7	Elbow extension, Wrist flexion	
	Tricecps, Wrist flexors	
C8	Ulnar deviation, Thumb extension,	
	Ulnar deviators, Thumb extensors	
T1	No weakness	
	Abduction little finger	
T2	No weakness	
	Finger intrinsics	
T3 – T12	No weakness	
L1	Hip flexion	
	Psoas	
L2	Hip flexion/Adduction/Medial rotation	
	Psoas, Hip adductors	

Contd...

Contd...

Nerve Root	Myotome	Patient Response
L3	Leg/Knee extension Psoas, quadriceps, thigh	
L4	Ankle dorsi flexion Tibialis anterior, Extensor hallucis	
L5	Great/Big toe extension Extensor hallucis, Peroneals	
S1	Knee flexion-Ankle plantar flexion/Foot eversion Harmstrings, Peroneals, Plantar flexors	
S2	Same as S1 except peroneals	
S3	None	
S4	Bladder, rectum	

14
Annexure

Assessment of Posture

PLUMB ALIGNMENT				
Front view: Deviated (Rt/Lt)		Back view: Deviated (Rt/Lt)		
Side view:				

SEGMENTAL ALIGNMENT				
Feet	Hammer Toes	Hallux Valgus	Low Ant Arch	Ant. Foot Varus
	Pronated	Supinated	Flat Long Arch	Pigeon Toes
Knees	Med. Rot	Lat. Rot	Knock Knees	
	Hyper Extent	Flexed	Bow Legs	Tibial Torsion
Pelvis	Leg in Adduct	Rotation	Tilt	Deviation
L. Back	Lordosis	Flat	Kyphosis	Scoliosis
U. Back	Kyphosis	Flat	Scap. Abducted	Scap. Elevated
Thorax	Depressed Chest	Elevated Chest	Rotation	Deviation
Spine	Total Curve	Lumbar	Thoracic	Cervical
Abdomen	Protruding	Scars	Antr. Tilt	Postr. Tilt
Shoulder	Low	High	Forward	Backward
Head	Forward	Torticolis	Lateral Tilt	Rotation

TESTS FOR FLEXIBILITY AND MUSCLE LENGTH			Rt	SHOE CORRECTION	Lt
Forward Bending:				Inner Wedge (Wide Heel)	
Trunk Extension:				(Narrow Heel)	
Trunk Side Bending:	Rt	Lt:		Level Heel Raise	
Tensor Fas Lata:	Rt	Lt:		Metatarsal Support	
Hip Flexors:	Rt	Lt:		Longitudinal Support	
Arm elevation:	Rt	Lt:		Notes:	

Rt	MUSCLE STRENGTH TESTS	Lt
	Mid, Low Trapezieus	
	Back Extensors	
	Gluteus Medius and Maximus	
	Harmstrings	
	Hip Flexors	
	Tibialis Posterior	

15
Annexure

Assessment of Gait

Observational Gait Analysis

Segment	Deviation	HS		FF		MST		HO		TO		ACC		MSW		DEC	
		R	L	R	L	R	L	R	L	R	L	R	L	R	L	R	L
Ankle	None																
Sagittal Plane	Foot flat																
	Foot slap																
	Heel off																
	No Heel off																
	Excess Plantar flexion																
	Excess Dorsi flexion																
	Toe drag																
	Toe clawing																
	Vaulting (Contralateral)																
Frontal Plane	Varus																
	Valgus																
Knee	None																
Sagittal Plane	Excess Flexion																
	Limited Flexion																
	No Flexion																
	Hyper Extension																
	Genu Recurvatum																
	Diminished Extension																
Frontal Plane	Varum																
	Valgum																
Hip	None																
Sagittal Plane	Excessive Flexion																
	Limited Flexion																
	No Flexion																
	Diminished Extension																
Frontal Plane	Abduction, Adduction																
	Ext. Rotation																
	Int. Rotation																
	Circumduction																
	Hiking																

Contd...

Contd...

		\multicolumn{14}{c	}{Observational Gait Analysis}
Segment	Deviation	\multicolumn{2}{c	}{HS}	\multicolumn{2}{c	}{FF}	\multicolumn{2}{c	}{MST}	\multicolumn{2}{c	}{HO}	\multicolumn{2}{c	}{TO}	\multicolumn{2}{c	}{ACC}	\multicolumn{2}{c	}{MSW}	\multicolumn{2}{c	}{DEC}
Pelvis	None	R	L	R	L	R	L	R	L	R	L	R	L	R	L	R	L
Sagittal Plane	Anterior Tilt																
	Posterior Tilt																
	Inc. Back. Rotation																
	Inc. Forward. Rotation																
	Lim. Back. Rotation																
	Lim. Forward. Rotation																
	Drops on Contralateral																
Trunk	None																
	Backward Rotation																
	Lateral lean																
	Forward Rotation																
	Backward Lean																
	Forward lean																

16 Annexure

Assessment of Functional Activity

SHORT MUSCULOSKELETAL FUNCTIONAL ASSESSMENT (SMFA)

These questions are about how much difficulty you may be having this week with your daily activities because of your injury or arthritis.

	Not at all Difficult	A Little Difficult	Moderately Difficult	Very Difficult	Unable to Do
1. How difficult is it for you to get in or out of a low chair?	☐	☐	☐	☐	☐
2. How difficult is it for you to open medicine bottles or jars?	☐	☐	☐	☐	☐
3. How difficult is it for you to shop for groceries or other things?	☐	☐	☐	☐	☐
4. How difficult is it for you to climb stairs?	☐	☐	☐	☐	☐
5. How difficult is it for you to make tight fist?	☐	☐	☐	☐	☐
6. How difficult is it for you to get in or out of the bath tub or shower?	☐	☐	☐	☐	☐
7. How difficult is it for you to get comfortable to sleep?	☐	☐	☐	☐	☐
8. How difficult is it for you to bend or kneel down?	☐	☐	☐	☐	☐
9. How difficult is it for you to use buttons snaps, hooks, or zippers?	☐	☐	☐	☐	☐
10. How difficult is it for you to cut your own finger nails?	☐	☐	☐	☐	☐
11. How difficult is it for you to dress yourself?	☐	☐	☐	☐	☐
12. How difficult is it for you to walk?	☐	☐	☐	☐	☐
13. How difficult is it for you to get moving after you have been sitting or lying down?	☐	☐	☐	☐	☐
14. How difficult is it for you to go out by yourself?	☐	☐	☐	☐	☐
15. How difficult is it for you to drive?	☐	☐	☐	☐	☐
16. How difficult is it for you to clean yourself after going to the bathroom?	☐	☐	☐	☐	☐
17. How difficult is it for you to turn knobs or levers	☐	☐	☐	☐	☐
18. How difficult is it for you to write or type?	☐	☐	☐	☐	☐
19. How difficult is it for you to pivot?	☐	☐	☐	☐	☐
20. How difficult is it for you to do your usual physical recreational activities?	☐	☐	☐	☐	☐
21. How difficult is it for you to do your usual leisure activities?	☐	☐	☐	☐	☐
22. How much difficulty are you having with sexual activity?	☐	☐	☐	☐	☐
23. How difficult is it for you to do light house work or yard work?	☐	☐	☐	☐	☐
24. How difficult is it for you to do heavy house work or yard work?	☐	☐	☐	☐	☐
25. How difficult is it for you to do your usual work?	☐	☐	☐	☐	☐

These next questions ask how often you are experiencing problems this week because of your injury or arthritis.

Contd...

Contd...

	None of the time	A Little of the time	Some of the time	Most of the time	All of the time
26. How often do you walk with a limp?	☐	☐	☐	☐	☐
27. How often do you avoid using your painful limbs or back?	☐	☐	☐	☐	☐
28. How often does your leg lock or give-way?	☐	☐	☐	☐	☐
29. How often do you have problems with concentration?	☐	☐	☐	☐	☐
30. How often does doing too much in one day affect what you do the next day?	☐	☐	☐	☐	☐
31. How often do you act irritable toward those around you?	☐	☐	☐	☐	☐
32. How often are you tired?	☐	☐	☐	☐	☐
33. How often do you feel disabled?	☐	☐	☐	☐	☐
34. How often do you feel angry or frustrated That you have this injury or arthritis?	☐	☐	☐	☐	☐

These questions are about how much you are bothered by problems you are having this week because of your injury or arthritis.

	Not at all Bothered	A Little Bothered	Moderately Bothered	Very Bothered	Unable Bothered
35. How much you are bothered by problems using your hands, arms, or legs?	☐	☐	☐	☐	☐
36. How much are you bothered by problems using your back?	☐	☐	☐	☐	☐
37. How much are you bothered by problems doing work around your home?	☐	☐	☐	☐	☐
38. How much are you bothered by problems With bathing, toileting dressing or other personal care?	☐	☐	☐	☐	☐
39. How much you are bothered by problems with sleep and rest?	☐	☐	☐	☐	☐
40. How much are you bothered by problems with leisure or recreational activities?	☐	☐	☐	☐	☐
41. How much are you bothered by problems with your friends, family or other important people in your life?	☐	☐	☐	☐	☐
42. How much are you bothered by problems with thinking, concentrating, or remembering?	☐	☐	☐	☐	☐
43. How much are you bothered by problems adjusting, or coping with your injury or arthritis?	☐	☐	☐	☐	☐
44. How much are you bothered by problems doing your usual work?	☐	☐	☐	☐	☐
45. How much are you bothered by problems with feeling dependent on others?	☐	☐	☐	☐	☐
46. How much are you bothered by problems with stiffness and pain?	☐	☐	☐	☐	☐

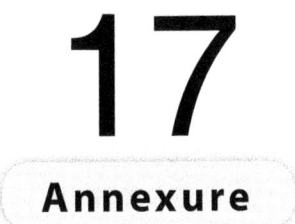

Assessment of Environment

Independent: The person receives no help with any of the behavioral components involved in the activity.

10. **No Assistance:** The person completes the activity without taking an inappropriate amount of time, without using assistance devices(s) or aid(s), without changing the environmental context, and without risking personal safety or well – being.

    Modified Independent: The person receives no help with any of the behavioral components involved in the activity. The person completes the activity independently but either takes an inappropriate amount of time, uses an assistive device(s) or aid(s), changes (or causes some one else to change) the environmental context or risks personal safety or wellbeing.

9. **Additional time:** The person completes the activity independently and safely but takes an inappropriate amount of time. At least one of the following is true. The person hesitates, makes repeated attempts, takes at least double the amount of time normally required to complete the activity.

8. **Assistive device:** The person completes the activity independently and safely by using an assistive device(s) or aids(s). The person may or may not take an inappropriate amount of time.

7. **Modified environment:** The person completes the activity independently and safely after changing (or causing some one else to change) the environmental context. The person may or may not take an inappropriate amount of time and may or may not use an assistive device(s) or aid(s).

6. **Safety considerations:** Either the person completes the activity independently with some risk to personal safety or well-being or the actions of another person present indicate that something about the activity poses a hazard. The person may or not take an inappropriate amount of time, may or may not use an assistive device(s) or aid(s) and may or may not change (or cause someone else to change) the environmental context.

    Modified Dependent: The person requires and receives help in the form of either supervision or physical assistance with at least one of the behavioral components involved in the activity. The person nevertheless contributes at least half (50–100%) of the total effort expended to complete the activity.

5. **Supervision or setup:** The person requires and receives help that only involves supervision (e.g., standing by, cueing, coaxing, setting up needed items or applying orthosis) i.e, no physical contact with a helper occurs during completion of the activity. The person contributes to all (100%) of the effort expended to complete the activity.

4. **Minimal contact assistance:** The person requires and receives assistance that involves physical contact with a helper during completion of activity. The person contributes nearly all (75–99%) of the effort expended to complete the activity.

3. **Moderate assistance:** The person requires and receives help that involves physical contact with a helper during completion of activity. The person still contributes most (50–74%) of the effort expended to complete the activity.

    Dependent:
    The person requires and receives help in the form of physical assistance with at least one of the behavioral components involved in the activity. Either the person contributes less than half (0% to 49%) of the effort expended to complete the activity or the activity is not completed.

2. **Maximal assistance:** The person contributes some (25–49%) of the effort expended to complete the activity.

1. **Total assistance:** The person contributes little or none (0–24%) of the effort expended to complete the activity.

0. **Activity not completed:** The person either is unable to complete the activity even with total assistance or declines to perform the activity.

18
Annexure

Assessment of Cranial Nerves

Cranial Nerve Examination

Nerve	Procedure	Patient Response
Olfactory	Assess the sense of smell with common odors.	
Optic	Visual acuity, Peripheral vision, Visual fields.	
	Corneal light reflex, Pupillary size and shape.	
Occulomotor	Assess the eye field deviation.	
	Pupillary light reflex test, Accommodation reflex test.	
Trochlear	Ask to turn adducted eye downwards.	
Trigeminal	Forehead, cheek, chin, sensation test	
	Corneal reflex test, Ask to clench jaws against resistance	
Abducent	Ask to turn the eye outwards.	
Facial	Facial expression testing, Eyebrow rising, Show teeth and smile.	
	Close the eyes tightly, Puff cheeks, Test sweet, salty, sour, bitter.	
Vestibulocochlear	Assess the balance, Eye-head coordination, Nystagmus	
	Weber's test: conduction, Rinner's test: sensorineural	
Glassopharyngeal	Assess the sweet, salt, sour, bitter on posterior one-third of tongue.	
	Gag reflex test.	
Vagus	Assess phonation and articulation, See movements of soft palate.	
	Swallowing, Pharyngeal sensation test.	
Spinal Accessory	Assess the strength of sternocleidomastoid and trapezius muscle.	
Hypoglossal	Assess the strength of the tongue movements, Tongue protrusion.	

19 Annexure

Assessment of Disease Specific Scale

STROKE:
- American Heart Association stroke outcome classification scale
- Arm Motor Ability Test
- Box and Block test
- Fugl-Meyer
- Lateropulsion Scale for Stroke
- Lower Extremity Motor Coordination Test
- Modified BBS for Stroke
- Modified MAS
- Ranking Scale
- Rivermaid Mobility Index
- Sodring Motor Evaluation of Stroke
- Trunk Control Test
- Trunk Impairment Scale
- Wolf Motor Function Test

SPINAL CORD INJURY:
- ASIA
- FIM for Spinal Cord Injuries
- Walking Index for Spinal Cord Injury
- Quadriplegic Index of Function
- Capabilities or Upper Extremity Test

PARKINSONS DISEASE:
- Dyskinesia Rating Scale
- Parkinson's Disease Questionnaire
- Hoehn and Yahr Classificatin of Disability Scale
- Unified Hunting Disease Rating Scale
- UPDRS

COMA SCALE:
- GCS
- Coma Recovery Scale
- Glasgow Outcome Scale
- Glasgow Epilepsy Outcome Scale
- Western Neurosensory Stimulation Profile

TRAUMATIC BRAIN INJURY:
- Glasgow Coma Scale
- RLA
- Glasgow Outcome Scale
- FIM

20 Annexure

Assessment of Primitive Reflex

Level	Reflex	Grade
Spinal Cord	Flexor withdrawal	
	Extensor thrust	
	Crossed extension	
	Palmar grasp	
	Plantar grasp	
	Sucking refex	
	Startle reflex	
	Rooting	
	Primitive walking	
Brainstem	STNR	
	ATNR	
	Tonic labyrinthine reflex	
	+ve and –ve supporting reaction	
Cortical	Equilibrium reaction in supine	
	Equilibrium reaction in prone	
	Equilibrium reaction in kneeling	
	Equilibrium reaction in sitting	
	Equilibrium reaction in standing	
Mid Brain	Optical rightening	
	Labyrinthine	
	Body on neck	
	Body on body	
	Neck rightening reaction	
Automatic	Moro reflex	
	Gallant trunk incurvatum	
	Landau's reflexes	
	Parachute reflexes	

Grade: 0: Absent
1: Tone Change: Slight transient with no movement of extremity.
2: Visible movements of the extremity.
3: Exaggerated full movement of the extremity.
4: Obligatory and sustained movement, lasting for more than 30 seconds.

21 Annexure

Assessment of Birth History

PRE-NATAL HISTORY

- Information on Pregnancy, any abortion, miscarriage or stillbirth.
- Systemic illness during pregnancy-Cardiac disease, Renal failure, Eclampsia.
- Exposure to toxins, alcohol, drugs like thalidomide.
- Acute maternal illness, Trauma, Radiation exposure.
- Family history and familial diseases.
- Fathers age and Mothers age during conception.
- Other siblings,
- Consanguinity.

NATAL HISTORY

- Information about breech delivery, umbilical cord strangulation, forceps delivery, delayed labour, cesarean delivery, vacuum used, meconium stained liquor.
- Term of Delivery
- Labour Pain
- Type of Delivery
- Place of Delivery
- Birth Trauma
- Condition of mother at the time of delivery.

POST-NATAL HISTORY

- Information about delivery type, Apgar score, Birth weight, premature birth, Birth cry.
- Jaundice, Neonatal sepsis, cranial malformations, metabolic causes (Hypocalcaemia, Hypernatremia).
- Intake of drugs like optin, valparin.

22

Annexure

Assessment of Milestone

Milestone Examination		
Milestone	Age Range	Achieved Age
Recognition of Mother	2-3 months	
Head Control	2-4 months	
Rolling Supine to Side Lying	2-4 months	
Rolling Supine to Prone	5-7 months	
Rolling Prone to Supine	5-7 months	
Sitting with Support	5-6 months	
Sitting without Support	7-9 months	
Transfers object one hand to the other	5-7 months	
Beginning Quadripod	7-9 months	
Crawling	8-10 months	
Beginning Pull to Standing	7-9 months	
Standing with Support	8-10 months	
Standing without Support	10-11 months	
Fine Motor Examination		
Hand grasp reflex	Birth - 5 months	
Visual regard	Birth - 2 months	
Swipes with whole hand	2-3 months	
Visually directed reaching	3-5 months	
Midline clasping of hands	2-5 months	
Reaches out to grasp object	4-5 months	
Plays with feet; bangs objects together	5 months	
Crude palming, ulnar fingers predominating	5-7 months	
Transfers object one hand to the other	6 months	
Lateral scissors grasp	8-9 months	
Pincer grasp, forefinger and thumb in opposition	10-11 months	
Poking and prodding with index finger	10-11 months	
Holds crayon	11 months	
Beginning voluntary release	11 months	
Precision grasp with fine pincer and controlled release	15 months	
Scribbles on paper	15-18 months	
Holds paper with other hand when scribbling	18 months	
Puts object in container and dumps contents	18 months	
Builds tower of three cubes	18 months	
Turns pages of book, perhaps two or three at time	21 months	
Unscrews jar lid	24 months	
Builds tower with eight cubes	30 months	

23
Annexure

Assessment of Paediatric Muscle Strength

Infants 1–2 years		Toddlers 2-5 years	
Activity	Grade	Activity	Grade
In prone		Squatting:	
Swimming:		Low kneel to high kneel:	
Rolling prone to supine:		High kneel to half-kneel:	
Reciprocal crawling:		Side step:	
Modified four-point kneeling		Standing on one foot:	
Reciprocal creeping:		Jumping from two feet:	
In supine		Jumping off a step:	
Hands to feet:		Toe walking:	
Rolling supine to prone with rotation		Heel-walking:	
In sitting		Tandem-walking:	
Pull to sit:		Stair –walking –upstairs:	
Sitting with propped arms:		Stair –walking –downstairs:	
Sitting without arm support- unsustained:		Ball throwing –overhead:	
Dynamic sitting without arm support –sustained:		Ball throwing- one handed:	
		Prehension –palmar supinate:	
In standing		Prehension –digital pronate:	
Supported standing:		Static tripod:	
Pulls to stand, stands with support:		Dynamic tripod:	
Side- step cruising:			
Controlled lowering with support:			
Stands without support:			
Stands from modified squat:			
Walk alone:		Impression:	

Functional: (F) Normal for age or only slight impairment or delay

Weak Functional: (WF) Moderate impairment or delay that affects activity pattern, base of support, or control against gravity, or decreases functional exploration

Non-Functional: (NF) Severe impairment or delay, activity pattern has only elements of correct muscular activity.

No-Function: Cannot do any function

24 Annexure

Assessment of Nutritional Status

Number of meals taken daily :
Protein intake :
Dairy product per day :
Legumes per week/day :
Eggs per week/day :
Meat, fish or poultry per week/day :
Consumption of fruits and vegetables per day :
Fluid intake :
Weight changes :
Has food intake decline in past three years :
Reasons for reduced intake :
Any loss of appetite :
Reduced taste/smell :
Any chewing, swallowing or problem in digestion :
Any other reason (e.g. dentures) :
Who prepared the food? :
Mode of feeding :
Unable to eat without assistance :
Self-fed with some difficulty :
Self-fed without any problem :
In comparison with other people of the same age, do they consider their,

Not as good/Do not know/As good/Better

EU GSPR Authorised Reprsentative
Logos Europe, 9 rue Nicolas Poussin
1700, La Rochelle, France
Phone: +33 (0) 6 67 93 73 78
E-mail: contact@logoseurope.eu

www.ingramcontent.com/pod-product-compliance
Ingram Content Group UK Ltd.
Pitfield, Milton Keynes, MK11 3LW, UK
UKHW050132170426
5217IPUK00051BA/1752